HEALTH-CARE
AND THE CHURCH:
A SHARED FOCUS

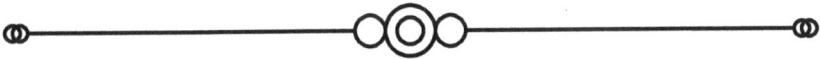

HEALTH-CARE AND THE CHURCH: A SHARED FOCUS

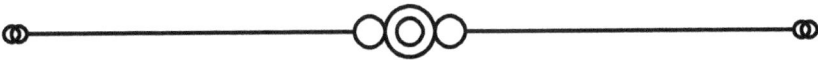

Phyllis C. Riles

Dedication:

To my amazing, selfless husband, Elder James Riles. "I love you more!" Thank you for all you are in my life and for all that you do!

To the best adult children and grandchildren, a mother could ever have. Thank you so much for always being so supportive of me— always!

To "the least of these." May your prosperity, health, and wellness arise through the ministry of the Church!

Table of Contents

Preface

"Father Abraham has many sons; many sons has Father Abraham. I am one of them, and so are you! So, let's just praise the Lord...."

I f you have ever attended Sunday School or Vacation Bible School (VBS), you probably could hum the tune along with those words. We learned early about Father Abraham and God's promises to him and his seed—his offspring. God promised that He would multiply Abraham's seed as much as the stars of the heavens. He also promised blessings upon blessings. Among those blessings is deliverance from sin and sickness and disease.

Health and healing are a significant part of the covenant promises between Abraham and God—a covenant which extends to us as Believers in the Lord Jesus Christ. We find the evidence of His unfailing CARE through us as the Church: His spiritual Body on the earth.

There is a sense of unity and safety in the community of Believers. I have experienced this countless times in my life. In 1986, for example, I was pregnant with my second child. On a Spring Sunday afternoon in the middle of Service, I went into full-blown, patterned breathing labor. As I was wheeled out of the church to go to the hospital, I recall the congregation erupting into cheers of support and excitement. After prayer for a safe delivery, I was taken to the hospital and, not long after, delivered a bouncing 5.5-pound baby boy. The sense of protection I felt from their prayers and support, coupled with a complete lack of fear, was comforting. After all, everyone has heard of someone giving birth someplace other than at the "hospital."

What if that experience could be translated to other areas of healthcare awareness? Is it possible that the church could be a hub for healthcare or possibly healthcare coordination for the community? How comforting could it be for persons with chronic heart disease to know that their community of Believers understood how to address their concerns and how to support them through education as well as prayer?

The purpose of this book is to set forward such considerations. I will not discuss medicines or medical procedures. Those are highly subjective and personal matters which should only be discussed with your health practitioner in the context of professional counsel. However, I sincerely hope that as you read this book, you will be inspired to explore God's covenant promises and discover how Health—CARE and the Church have a shared focus. It is a focus that you can help fine-tune through your own involvement as you choose to be the Church in motion.

Foreword

The urgency created by the COVID-19 crisis in 2020 suddenly made the topic of disease prevention and treatment a household discussion. Everyone had questions and concerns. National lockdowns and restrictions affected all of us. The impact hit hard, fueled by a fear factor due to confusing or conflicting information and misconceptions about proceeding forward. No one had a reference point for the implications of a worldwide pandemic. Countries blocked their borders, businesses shut down, leaving people unemployed, and churches closed their doors in response.

My husband Bishop Kevin Dickerson and I remained directly engaged to stabilize people who grappled with often debilitating blows from sickness, death, as well as the fear and depression produced by loss and isolation. As my husband often says, "Shepherds should smell like sheep." In other words, we are to be touched by what touches them. We don't observe their pain or struggles from afar; we enter their experiences with them, bringing the love, wisdom, and comfort of God into their situations.

Through the years, we have had our own questions and discussions about how to help and heal the hurting while taking measures to keep people safe. As a Bishop over several churches, my husband has spent countless hours in prayer and research to help those under his leadership navigate the unprecedented path ahead.

Although many seem to have lost their way during these difficult and confusing times, the Church cannot lose its voice or influence. The gospel we proclaim exalts Jesus Christ, who saves, heals, and delivers

(John 3:16; Acts 10:38). Scripture is clear that God wants people to be healthy in body and soul **(3 John 1:2).** The covenant God cut with His people when He delivered them from Egypt included instructions to ensure their health, with the promises that He would "put none of these diseases" upon them **(Exodus 15:26).** For this reason, I am very pleased by the subject of Phyllis C. Riles' timely and instructive new book: Health—CARE and the Church: A Shared Focus.

Phyllis Carter-Riles, RN, is the founder of Phyllis C. Riles Consulting. It is a healthcare consultancy designed to bridge the gap between healthcare and Kingdom CARE through education, strategy, and camaraderie. Leveraging her Bachelor of Science in Nursing and Master of Health Administration degrees, Phyllis uses her more than thirty years of nursing experience to promote health through innovative and insightful topics. In Irving, Texas, she began the Rapha Health Ministry for our church—Dayspring Family Church. Here, she developed programs such as "Walking by Faith," which brought women together weekly to walk while singing, praying, and exercising. She taught CPR classes for our church and conducted a Church Disinfection Seminar for our Vision Fellowship, the group of churches that my husband serves as Bishop over. Phyllis applies process improvement principles to create programs that benefit the Church and the healthcare system as a certified Six-Sigma Yellow Belt.

Phyllis is a board-certified leader in the arena of infection control. Her experience in all levels of obstetric nursing, including management and education, makes her uniquely suited to present health care principles and complex science in an easily relatable format to those of us in the general, non-medical public.

But even more importantly, as the self-described "Kingdom Nurse," Phyllis understands the mission of the Church, as well as the challenges that confront it. With clarity and insight, she illuminates compelling

Scriptural truths to inspire you to view health care through the lens of the Great Commission. And, through her gift of storytelling, when she describes how her medical qualifications positioned her to "be" the Church to someone in need, you will surely confront your own beliefs as you evaluate the opportunities before you to act with measurable results.

I have known Phyllis for more than 20 years, as she has served God, our congregation, and others with excellence and compassion. I can attest to the strength of her ability to educate and elevate mindsets in a way that resonates with those who hear her. I hope that as you read this book, you will gain either a new or a freshly ignited passion for sharing the focus of healthcare and kingdom care. If you are a member of the Church—the Body of Christ—it is my prayer that you will awaken to your role to be His heart and hands extended to reach into every man's world to "be" the Church...especially to "the least of these."

Dr. Sonjia Dickerson
Dayspring Family Church, Executive Pastor and Overseer
American Heart Association, Ambassador and Panel Contributor

Introduction

Have you ever heard the phrases "the church is a hospital for the saints" or "the saints' live with what kills everyone else?" Growing up in the church, it seemed silly to me, but what most adults said didn't make sense to us when we were kids, did it? Fortunately for me, the revelation of these sayings became obvious the older I became.

These statements were a declaration of hope! The woman with the issue of blood proved this hope when she pressed in to get to Jesus despite all cultural and societal reasons that she shouldn't. She knew in Him she would finally find what she so desperately needed: healing. I can imagine that she tried to make herself invisible because she was not supposed to be outside among people in her condition. Ignoring the jeers of those who saw her, she made her way to Jesus through the crowds, telling herself if I could just touch the hem of His clothes, I would be made whole.

Consider her story:

"And a certain woman, which had an issue of blood twelve years, And had suffered many things of many physicians, and had spent all that she had, and was nothing bettered, but rather grew worse, When she had heard of Jesus, came in the press behind, and touched his garment, for she said, If I may touch but his clothes, I shall be whole. And straightway the fountain of her blood was dried up; and she felt in her body that she was healed of that plague. And Jesus, immediately knowing in himself that virtue had gone out of him, turned him about in the press, and said, Who touched my clothes?

And his disciples said unto him, Thou seest the multitude thronging thee, and sayest thou, Who touched me? And he looked round about to see her that had done this thing. But the woman fearing and trembling, knowing what was done in her, came and fell down before him, and told him all the truth. And he said unto her, Daughter, thy faith hath made thee whole; go in peace, and be whole of thy plague (Mark 5:25-34)."

It is not hard to imagine that this unnamed woman suffered physically, mentally, and socially through those twelve years. The Bible even clues us in on the financial impact that it had on her as well. It does not tell us if she had a family, but one can guess that she may have. Imagine the emotional toll her illness must have taken on her family as well. Living with someone who was barred from society and from performing the duties of a woman because she was considered unclean could not have been easy for them either..

How many people today are suffering and isolated like that woman? The complexities of her circumstances carry painful similarities to situations people face today. And the Church, the Body of Christ in the earth, is appointed to be light and salt **(see Matthew 5:13-16)** for the benefit of all we may encounter in need.

The focus on health in the Church is multifactorial. It is as extensive and varied as the people.

> "
> Preparations to minister to the community's health start with first realizing that health and wellness are two of the Church's main goals"

The health of the people is a significant focus for the Kingdom of God.

What is Health?

What is health? Dr. Andrija Štampar, a prominent scholar from Croatia in social medicine and public health and one of the founders of the World Health Organization (WHO), proposed a definition in 1948. This generally accepted definition states that "health is a state of complete physical, mental, and social well-being and not merely the absence of disease or infirmity" [1].

Because of life experiences and maturity, I now know the significance of coming to the House of God when one is ill. For it is there that one will meet Jesus, and it is there that one will receive the word that they need, go in peace, and be made whole.

Since the days before Jesus showed up as the embodiment of the will of God in motion, the temple was the place where healing was proclaimed. The priests served this function and figuratively, in some cases, still do. In this book, we will journey through the revelation of God as Healer and His plan that His Church—the Body of Christ—is the instrument of it. We will also discuss how the modern-day church has a responsibility concerning the health of God's people—spirit, soul, and body. We will also provide actionable suggestions on how it can demonstrate that focus in a day and time when it is needed the most.

Let's Pray: *Father, in the name of Jesus, we ask You to guide us as we take this journey towards enlightenment of health—CARE. Please help us understand how to CARE for one another as You so deeply care for us. Open our eyes and hearts to the possibilities to serve Your people that we have never considered before. We realize that we are Your hands and feet in the earth. Give us the desire and the know-how to make You proud as we carry out every assignment that You have placed within our hearts that link directly to Your heart for Your people. As we learn of these opportunities, we thank You for the necessary provisions to bring them to pass. Amen!*

How Do You Treat the Least of These?

Chapter I

My nursing career began in Labor and Delivery. I was blessed to work in a specialty area that didn't always take new graduate nurses. I was able to help bring new life into families. I am still proud of this time in my career. In many instances, next to the doctor, I was the first person to hold the newly born babies and welcome them into the world. What an honor!

I have occupied several leadership roles throughout my career. One incident marked me forever when I was in the role of Educator for the Women's Services department for my hospital. I'd like to share that with you. At that time, my office was located down the hall from the Labor and Delivery unit. I had been an L & D nurse for many years. On that day, I was asked to leave my office work to care for a unique situation with a laboring patient. The report I was given was remarkable indeed. She was a forensic patient. A "forensic patient" is one under arrest. This patient was incarcerated in prison, not merely in jail—but also was pregnant and being induced to deliver her full-term baby. Another important thing about her was that her baby would be placed with a family member, put into the foster care system, or possibly even adopted out right away. I'll call her "Ann."

Ann

Ann was reportedly a dangerous person. She was shackled to the bed and flanked by two armed guards who were always physically present in the room. One of the guards was male. Ann was a "bad girl." All the nurses were afraid and were worried about being assigned to care for her. We didn't know what Ann had done. It was against the rules to ask. It was at this point that I was brought into the story.

When I walked into her room, Ann greeted me first.

"Hey, sister," she said with a big smile.

My response to her was "Hey, sister," with a smile that met hers. We bonded instantly. We laughed and as we talked throughout her labor. I took care of her as her body prepared to bring her innocent baby into the world. It was possible that Ann's baby would never know its birth mother. I coached Ann through her contractions. I used therapeutic touch and the other labor management techniques that I had used more times than I could remember. I humanized Ann as she acted like all the other hundreds of women I had taken care of in my career did when they were in labor. It was painful. She needed someone to reassure her that she was doing a good job and it would be okay. At that moment, I was her family. I was her support.

As the contractions became increasingly more uncomfortable, I asked Ann, "Would you like to listen to some music while you labor?"

She said, "Yes."

I went to my office and got my cassette radio player.

When I returned, I asked her what she wanted to listen to. She said, "Whatever you want to hear." She always looked me straight in my eyes when we spoke—like old friends. I put on a gospel CD. It seemed to help her to relax. Considering the circumstances, she was my friend, and I wanted to help her have the best experience possible.

A Labor of Love

I served her like I had my so many other patients. I advocated for her to get an epidural once the contractions became too much for her to manage. In the 21st century, women don't have to suffer in pain during childbirth unless they want an all-natural birth. Ann wasn't a first-time mom, and she delivered relatively quickly. She chose not to see her baby. But I did. I whispered "Jesus is Lord" in her little ears as I had done so many times to newborns before. If they never heard it again, they would at least have heard it once. I believed their little spirits would rejoice because they knew it was true.

Ann's baby went to the nursery, and the next day, she went back to prison. As I recall meeting her, tears run down my face even now. I had been allowed to show the love of God to one of "the least of these."

God's Grace

In the eyes of the others, Ann was no more than an animal, someone accursed and to be feared. According to the behavior of some, she didn't deserve to be treated with dignity and respect. After all, the word was she was "bad." She had two armed guards. Therefore, they felt she had to be an awful human being. But in my mind, the point was simply: Ann was a human and deserved to be treated as such with dignity.

I provided Ann with excellent care that day. But my human connection with her was more than excellent.

I was criticized for my bond with her, including playing music for her. Music therapy is a known strategy used as an alternative to help laboring women cope with the pain of contractions. Why didn't Ann deserve that? Did she not deserve to be taken care of using all the techniques that I knew? Did not Ann deserve to have relief from the anguish of the painful contractions? Did she not deserve a season of "emotional health?"

I quickly quieted the criticism. I was pleased and thankful for the opportunity to have made a difference in Ann's life that day. I believe by faith that she felt the love of the Father in me. I do not know what happened to Ann after our encounter in Labor and Delivery. But the memory of her touched me deeply. I am forever honored that God used me to show her His love. Ann experienced the Kingdom of God: Righteousness (God's ways of doing and being right), peace, and joy simply from being acknowledged as a person worthy of respect. That day while my hospital provided Ann healthcare, I demonstrated and engaged with her as the Church.

The Least of These

In Matthew 25:31,40, Jesus said: "When the Son of man shall come in his glory, and all the holy angels with him, then shall he sit upon the throne of his glory: And before him shall be gathered all nations: and he shall separate them one from another, as a shepherd divideth his sheep from the goats: And he shall set the sheep on his right hand, but the goats on the left. Then shall the King say unto them on his right hand, Come, ye blessed of my Father, inherit the kingdom prepared for you from the foundation of the world: For I was an hungred, and ye gave me meat: I was thirsty, and ye gave me drink: I was a stranger, and ye took me in: Naked, and ye clothed me: I was sick, and ye visited me: I was in prison, and ye came unto me. Then shall the righteous answer him, saying, Lord, when saw we thee an hungred, and fed thee? or thirsty, and gave thee drink? When saw we thee a stranger, and took thee in? or naked, and clothed thee? Or when saw we thee sick, or in prison, and came unto thee? And the King shall answer and say unto them

> " Verily I say unto you, Inasmuch as ye have done it unto one of the least of these my brethren, ye have done it unto me."

As strange as it may sound, some struggle with Christ's command to feed the hungry as though it is a tricky thing. Unfortunately, in this instance, people are really struggling with their own implicit biases. What is that? An implicit bias is a strong dislike for a group of people or a person that one holds without even being aware of it because it is subconscious. Many people struggle with feeding the hungry or giving to the person begging on the corner with a sign that says "Disabled vet. I am hungry." Why? It has been ingrained in us that we shouldn't eat if we don't work. We look at these people and what we think we see with our natural eyes is a man or a woman who is "able-bodied," and we assume that they should work. Often, we even think things like, "They just want the money to buy liquor or drugs." Why would I give them my hard-earned money?"

Matthew 25: 31-40 paints a picture of Jesus returning, and after having divided the sheep from the goats, He says to those on His right hand, come you blessed of my Father, inherit the kingdom that was prepared for you from the foundation of the world. There are many instances in the Bible where Jesus showed compassion for the poor. He could often be seen instructing His disciples to feed people. However, He never said, "They knew they were coming to this conference; they should have brought their lunch!" or "Look, I only have enough for me and my twelve. They should have prepared." No, instead, in this passage, we see that He was genuinely concerned with the hungry.

The Less Fortunate

As the Church, we also have obligations to the poor. Many churches have food pantries or days when they serve the homeless and less fortunate. Jesus demonstrates the importance of lending a helping hand to others when we are able. Many people keep spare change in their cars to give to people in need as they are prompted by the Holy Spirit. The Bible is clear in **Romans 15:1** that the strong are to bear the infirmities of the weak. It does not say "bear the infirmities of the weak as long as they are not responsible for the condition that they find themselves in."

In **Matthew 25:36-40,** Jesus described the actions of those whom He said never knew Him, when He said, "When I was in prison, you didn't visit me. We live in a society where people are cast away easily. Forgotten. Realistically, everyone is not called to be a prison minister, but we all can support someone who is. Better yet, we can all help someone who is imprisoned in their minds, in their circumstances, or in a state of hopelessness. Jesus is saying here, as His Church— His representatives on the earth—we are to care for each other as He would. I am sure that you have heard the saying, "We are the hands and feet of Jesus." We are to serve others like Him. He was a servant. He laid aside His deity to come in human flesh to experience our humanity. Jesus was very well in touch with who he was. He did not suffer from an identity crisis. He also knew what His mission was. He came to be the spotless sacrifice for men's sins. However, he also healed, delivered, and set captives free during that time.

During His ministry on earth, Jesus had many opportunities to challenge the norms and traditions of the culture. Jesus was faced with racism and separatism, just as we are today. But He refused to allow those things to keep Him from doing the work He was sent to do. He came for all men. Jesus said in **John 10:10, "The thief cometh not, but for to steal, and to kill, and to destroy: I am come that they might have life, and that they might have it more abundantly."**

Social, Economic, and Health Disparities

Social, economic, and health disparities are still commonplace in society across the globe. Research studies reveal that minorities, especially African Americans, are disproportionally marginalized across most spectrums of life in the United States. In 1966, during a press conference while at the convention of the Medical Committee on Human Rights in Chicago, Dr. Martin Luther King was quoted as saying, "Of all the forms of inequality, injustice in health is the most shocking and the most inhuman because it often results in physical death."[2] Unfortunately, the state of health in the United States is not much better than it was in the 1960s. In fact, in some instances it is worse.

Data collected by the Centers for Disease Control and Prevention (CDC) from a 2015 study showed that African Americans are living with diseases that are more common in people of older age groups. Additionally, they are more likely to die from any cause than their Caucasian counterparts.[3]

Healing the sick was one of Jesus' earthly ministries. **Acts 10:38 states, "How God anointed Jesus of Nazareth with the Holy Ghost and with power: who went about doing good and healing all that were oppressed of the devil; for God was with him."** Despite opposition from religious leaders and their traditions, Jesus said what He heard the Father speak to Him, and He did only what He saw the Father do. As a result, no one ever left His presence the same.

All who encountered Jesus left better physically, emotionally, and spiritually. Do you remember what He said that He came to do in **John 10:10**? He came to bring abundant life.

Segregation and racism were a part of life even in the time of Jesus. Let's consider the story of the Canaanite woman. She was not of the house of Israel. Jesus was sent to them at this point in His ministry. While it seems harsh, it illustrates how disparities can occur, but Jesus' ultimate response is what is notable in this instance.

"And, behold, a woman of Canaan came out of the same coasts, and cried unto him, saying, Have mercy on me, O Lord, thou son of David; my daughter is grievously vexed with a devil. But he answered her not a word. And his disciples came and besought him, saying, Send her away; for she crieth after us. But he answered and said, I am not sent but unto the lost sheep of the house of Israel. Then came she and worshipped him, saying, Lord, help me. But he answered and said, It is not meet to take the children's bread, and to cast it to dogs. And she said, Truth, Lord: yet the dogs eat of the crumbs which fall from their masters' table. Then Jesus answered and said unto her, O woman, great is thy faith: be it unto thee even as thou wilt. And her daughter was made whole from that very hour (Matthew 15:22-28)."

Jesus showed compassion for the woman and her daughter because of her great faith. She was healed immediately. He realized that she was not of the Jewish community, but she was a person with great faith in His ability to meet her need, which moved Him. It is our responsibility as the Church to be moved with compassion just as Jesus was.

As the Church, we can set people on the path to healing and wholeness.

" A kind word, a gesture of humanity, or even a smile can supply healing salve to the soul."

The development of a culture in the church that embraces the importance of achieving healthy lifestyles is essential.

We are to use our voices to speak up against injustices and disparities as they show up. The Bible tells us that we are to strengthen our brothers. Many people are suspicious and distrustful of the medical industry. Sadly, there are documented examples that validate their beliefs and distrust. Others simply do not have access to care. As the Church, the Body of Christ in the earth, what you can do to improve the disparities in care that minorities in your community experience. We also have the responsibility to use our influence to correct the wrongs in our society. We have voting power. Can you serve as a volunteer at a nonprofit organization or organize one if there isn't one that addresses these issues?

Search your heart. Do you hold implicit biases against groups of people—biases so ingrained in you that you were unaware of them? Do you avoid certain ethnic groups? Do you have preconceived notions about them? Ask God to reveal these biases to you. Repent as needed and turn away from those thoughts and feelings. Turn your back on them. Purpose in your heart to show the love of God in every area of your life, even to the "least of these."

Let's Pray: *Father, in Jesus' name. We thank You for Your love for all people, including the "least." Please forgive us for turning our eyes away when we see the less fortunate than us. Forgive us for operating in a spirit of judgementalism, looking down on others who don't look, act, or even smell like us. You gave us an example in Your Word of how Jesus CARED for everyone whether they were old or young, poor, or rich, sick, or well. Please give us Your heart for people. Give us a heart that would cause us to be selfless and to give freely as You have freely given to us. No longer, Father, will we get spiritual deafness when You prompt us to give to someone. No longer will we operate in a spirit of selective hearing when You give us Your word to give to someone that will bless and strengthen them for, we realize that it is not always money that You are prompting us to give. Let us not be slow to move when You prompt us to act, but we will operate as if You were standing there watching because You are. Give us keen and sharp ears as Your spirit speaks to us—the Church. In Jesus' name. Amen!*

The Kingdom of God-The Church

Chapter II

Healthcare has changed over the years. The provision of care has completely morphed over the decades since the beginning of modern medicine. We now have free-standing emergency rooms and telemedicine, where office visits are conducted entirely over the internet. We have added a specialized healthcare worker called the Nurse Practitioner (NP) to the medical workforce. The NP not only helps a doctor run their medical practice but can work independently in collaboration with a doctor and open their own clinic.

There are many ways the Church can share the focus for health in its communities. The Nurse Practitioner is an untapped resource in many underserved communities. Can you imagine a church that hosts a clinic a couple of times a week that is staffed by an NP for their members as well as people in the neighborhood? The goals that this would accomplish are limitless. Think of the number of people who would enter the church doors who might not otherwise. Not only could this be an opportunity to minister to them physically, but it would be a chance to share the life-changing good news of Jesus Christ as well. We will talk more about starting health-related services in later chapters.

From the start of my nursing career over 30 years ago, my desire was to educate God's people. I have taken advantage of every opportunity I have been given to speak, conduct classes, and host health care events, including blood drives at my church. I have always felt a responsibility for this. In all these years, that prompting—which some call a "burden" and others call an assignment—has not waned or altered. My call to minister to God's people physically and spiritually is the "cherry on the top" of an amazing nursing career. The healthcare industry and the church share a responsibility for helping people live healthy lives. Healthy people live naturally fulfilling lives and demonstrate Biblical health that positions them to walk out spiritually prosperous ones.

The Kingdom's Culture

It is impossible to discuss Biblical health and its connections to the Church without first establishing what the Kingdom of God is and is not. Used interchangeably with the Kingdom of Heaven, according to the King James Dictionary, the word kingdom corresponds with Strong's H4438.4 It means reign, royal power, dominion, rule. The Kingdom of God is not a physical location that you can navigate to by using your GPS. It is, however, just as real. More so, in fact.

The Pharisees questioned Jesus about the Kingdom of God, and His amazing response was full of revelation to those who have spiritual ears to hear then and now. **"And when he was demanded of the Pharisees, when the kingdom of God should come, he answered them and said, the kingdom of God cometh not with observation: Neither shall they say, Lo here! or, lo there! for, behold, the kingdom of God is within you" (Luke 17:20-21).**

If the Pharisees were modern-day men, they should have responded, "Wow, that's deep, Jesus! Explain more, please." But they didn't. Jesus has, however, explained more to us. God is the sovereign King, and

Jesus is the ruler. Because God is love, the Kingdom is all love. Let's say it like this: the Kingdom's culture is love.

Every city or town has a culture. I am from Chicago. It has a culture. Midwesterners, especially Chicagoans, while nice people, tend to be reserved at first meeting. The first time my husband and I drove to Chicago from Texas, we arrived after dark. My dear husband, born in Oklahoma and raised in Texas, has never met a stranger—never! I believe he seeks out strangers to talk to purposely. As we were getting our luggage out of the trunk of the car, a man came walking up the sidewalk minding his business. Piercing the darkness and the subsequent silence came the friendliest "How are you doing, sir?" from my husband. Our son and I looked at each other in wide-eyed disbelief. Both of us were thinking No! You don't speak to strangers here! Clueless, my husband shrugged at the lack of response from the man who had looked at him as if to say, Do I know you? Why are you talking to me? We finished getting our luggage and went into the house without incident. I don't think my husband understands the culture of the Midwest; he still speaks to strangers when we visit. In fact, I do, too, sometimes—just not in Chicago.

"
Yes, the Kingdom of God has a culture, and it is love!"

John 13:34-35 puts it this way: "A new commandment I give unto you, That ye love one another; as I have loved you, that ye also love one another. By this shall all men know that ye are my disciples, if ye have love one to another." It is the God kind of love, agape, that wants to see others do well. Obtaining and keeping health and healthy lifestyles is one way we do well.

Health and healing are often used synonymously, but they are not. Healing is a process that is undertaken to achieve health. It is necessary to rid the body of sickness, disease, and DIS-ease despite the type.

God made provision for the healing of humanity. **Isaiah 53:4-5** says, **"Surely he hath borne our griefs, and carried our sorrows: yet we did esteem him stricken, smitten of God, and afflicted. But he was wounded for our transgressions, he was bruised for our iniquities: the chastisement of our peace was upon him, and with his stripes, we are healed."**

As we discussed earlier, health is a state of well-being socially, mentally, and physically. Going forward, we will define health as the freedom from DIS- "ease." Britannica.com defines disease as "any harmful deviation from the normal structural or functional state of an organism."5

Let's break this down further. "DIS" according to Merriam-Webster. com, is "exclude, do the opposite, not"6 "Ease" is "comfortable, effortlessness, freedom of burden."7 It is peace, tranquility, calmness, enjoyment, repose, prosperity, contentment, and well-being, to name a few! Here is a good place for you to put your own definition of ease. What is that normal state of "ease" that God has created you to live in that the spirit of "dis" is coming to disrupt?

In **Romans 12**, the Bible describes our function as the Body of Christ: **"For as we have many members in one body, and all members have not the same office: So we, being many, are one body in Christ, and every one members one of another" (Romans 12:4-5).**

We have been given a responsibility to care for one another. The Word of God tells us to **"bear ye one another's burdens, and so fulfil the law of Christ (Galatians 6:2).** We are also to **"be kindly affectioned one** to another with brotherly love; in honor preferring one another" (Romans 12:10).

The "Church" Versus a Church

If you were to google the word "Church," you would immediately find a definition that refers to a building where people gather to worship a deity. While this is factual, it is not entirely true. But the biblical meaning of the word "Church" is far more substantial and significant than the mere brick and mortar of a building or the fabric of a tent.

The Greek word for Church is *ekklesia*. It refers to people or a group of people who have been called out of their homes into a public place, an assembly. This definition is based on the Greek Lexicon on the BibleStudyTools.com.[8] The word "Church" is much more than a physical building.

The Apostle Paul supplies clarity to the question of what the word "Church" is referring to. **"And he is the head of the body, the church: who is the beginning, the firstborn from the dead; that in all things he might have the preeminence"** (Colossians 1:18). Clearly, Paul is not referring to a building here. He lets us know that Jesus is the head of the body, the Church. To illuminate more, Jesus is the head of the body; we are the body, the Church.

The early Church embraced its role as a "group of people who have been called out" according to the definition of ekklesia.8 **"Then they that gladly received his word were baptized: and the same day there were added unto them about three thousand souls. And they continued steadfastly in the apostles' doctrine and fellowship, and in breaking of bread, and in prayers. And fear came upon every soul: and many wonders and signs were done by the apostles. And all that believed were together and had all things common; And sold their** possessions and goods, and parted them to all men, as every man had need" (Acts 2:40-45).

Churches do well in this area as it relates to the tangible giving to each other. Clothing drives and food give-a-ways are common. The Bible even encourages us to care for the widow and the orphan. We serve a God who gives unselfishly. He gave His only Son to redeem us back to Himself because sin had driven us apart. Therefore, with love as our motivation, we, the Church, are to give unselfishly to meet the needs of those around us who desperately hunger to be fed the truth of who God is and wants to be to them. **"Take heed therefore unto yourselves, and to all the flock, over the which the Holy Ghost hath made you overseers, to feed the church of God, which he hath purchased with his own blood" (Acts 20:28).**

Preparing church leadership for leading the congregation and its community is critical to growing and maintaining a healthy organization for the Kingdom. Having an assessment of the spiritual fortitude is extremely important as the church's mission, vision, and values are developed.

Mission, Visions, and Values

The mission, vision, and values are different than the doctrine. I know that sounds like business lingo. Winning souls is a business. It is Kingdom business. Having a mission, vision, and values statement flanked by strategy and goals/objectives supply a solid foundation for your organization.

A mission statement is the "why" your church exists. It describes your purpose for being an organization. The vision statement puts into words what the future state of your church will be based upon its "why." For instance, if the mission of your church is to bring the hope of Jesus Christ to a particular community that is downtrodden and marginalized, your vision could be to see "X" be the church of choice in the "Y" community where people find the light of hope through the power of God's love! The values are the beliefs or culture on which both the mission and vision stand. "X" church is the place where joy, peace, and love abide. Finally, the goals and objectives will help you measure how successful you were with the other elements.

We then put strategies in place to flesh out the missions, goals, and values. These are the details of your church. The strategies determine how you will execute your goals—the details such as whether you will have a school or a daycare. A key strategy might be to design and implement a senior citizen program because your church has a substantial elderly population. With a mission to reach that part of the population, and a goal to serve, let's say 100 seniors in 6 weeks, the strategy to create a senior citizen program¬—perhaps to help them with necessary errands or to provide groceries—would help accomplish that goal. Missions, goals, values, and strategies will combine to create a framework to mobilize members to reach the community and any mission field you may find.

In this fictitious church example, the community that you serve may be poor, have a significant number of teen pregnancies, and its residents have many health issues. Strategies around improving the health of this population could easily be evaluated depending on the measurable goals and objectives that were set. One goal could be to decrease the incidence of teenage pregnancy by 50 percent by developing a girl's self-esteem program that focuses on self-image, high school graduation, and career goals. This goal would be measured for success by determining if the benchmark of 50 percent was met.

Establishing a foundation upon spiritual equipment and gifting is as important as the mission, vision, and goal statement development, if not more. Figuring out and knowing the spiritual gifts of your team supports the development of those statements and the subsequent programs that come from them. You are probably saying that is a stretch. It isn't.

> "
> A church that focuses on the health of its community will find the use of these gifts invaluable."

A church that embraces the flow of the Spirit through the manifestation of the gifting of the people is powerful. It is in this power that the goals will be achieved. Not, may be, but will be achieved.

In the Bible, **Romans 12, Ephesians 4, and Corinthians 12** list the spiritual gifts that God through His spirit has provided to the church individually and thereby collectively. Mature Believers need to know what their gifts are and how they contribute to the strength—the health—of the Church body as a whole. Gifts of administration, the apostle, discernment, encourager/exhortation, evangelism, faith, giving, hospitality, help, healing, knowledge, leadership, pastor, prophecy, teaching, tongues, serving, showing mercy, and wisdom were given to edify. The church that has many of these gifts at work will be a force to be reckoned with. All of these will lead a congregation in reaching health in every area of life.

It is also critical that church leaders and other influential Christian leaders remember the power that their voices hold. The opinions released over the pulpit or across the internet carry great weight. Unfortunately, influential voices can promote misinformation or disinformation, which can be dangerous. Personal opinions must be kept personal, and only those things that have proven health-related value be shared publicly. Not everyone searches things out for themselves. Some will swallow whatever is said without verifying whether it is true or logically makes sense! This places even greater responsibility upon leadership for people to think, research, study, and pray through to their own solid beliefs and convictions.

Sister Sally

Sister Sally is a fabricated name I will use to represent several Believers who have followed her beliefs only to experience the same results.

Sister Sally was a strong Believer who loved God and His word. She found herself suffering from hypertension, aka high blood pressure. She first followed her doctor's advice, taking her medication as directed. Sister Sally then began following a group of Christian influencers whose medicine beliefs were different from hers. She soon began to modify her thought processes to align with what she perceived to be their beliefs and stopped taking her high blood pressure medication. Without her medication, her blood pressure continued to climb unbeknownst to her. Sister Sally suffered a massive stroke and passed away shortly thereafter.

Was the influence of the Christian leaders at fault for her decision to quit taking her medication? Of course, not. That would be difficult to prove. Frankly, they possibly had never spoken to her directly in all reality. However, we must be mindful of the power that our words carry and what the ramifications of them are when taken to heart. Medication can help people manage symptoms while they continue to make helpful adjustments that can result in better health and wholeness.

How then can a church aid with providing health education to its members without fearing someone taking what was said either out of context or literally? The provision of solid and correct information is essential. The Bible says in **Proverbs 4:7, "Wisdom is the principal thing; therefore, get wisdom: and with all thy getting get understanding."**

Providing high-level, official information is a great way to avoid the traps of giving advice that could be detrimental when over-generalized. Using health professionals in the congregation is an excellent way to use your voice in health matters without professionally stepping outside of one's expertise.

I caution about taking a stance on health issues using one's personal beliefs as a platform, but the role of the Pastor or other lay leaders is clear in the Bible. The Levitical priest held a critical position as it related to the health of the Israelites. **Leviticus 13** gives us a glimpse into the role of the priest as a health advisor, diagnostician, and the CDC as he dealt with people who were suspected of having leprosy. He was given specific details on diagnosing, isolating, and pronouncing them healed.

Can you imagine the weight of the responsibility the priest must have felt for his community? He not only had the life of the sick person in his hands, but he had the responsibility to protect the lives of others. Leprosy was highly contagious, with devastating effects if left untreated. I wonder how many times the priest envisioned the people he prayed for during the day when he closed his eyes at night. I wonder how often he thought of them when he should have been relaxing. Ministering to and healing the sick is important to God. James, the brother of Jesus, wrote in **James 5:14, "Is any sick among you? let him call for the elders of the church; and let them pray over him, anointing him with oil in the name of the Lord."**

> " The church that aligns itself with the will of God as it relates to the health of the people is a church that is positioned to provide undeniable value to the community"

While the pastor and other leaders won't be directly responsible for determining if someone is "unclean," they can help put resources in place to address the cause of their DIS-ease. One element of the needed resources is the physical building—the tent of meeting as it was called in the Old Testament.

Let's pray: *We thank You for the healing ministry of Your Son, Jesus! We are so grateful that You have given us Your Church to be at oneness with You. Thank You for the redemptive work of the cross. Thank You for the apostles, the prophets, the evangelists, the pastors, and teachers, to equip us for works of service so that the body of Christ may be built up until we all reach unity in the faith and in the knowledge of the Son of God and become mature, attaining to the whole measure of the fullness of Christ. Please show us how to walk through this life as representatives of You in everything we do. May our words release life, wealth, and health, and our actions inspire others to want to live for You. Father, thank You for the strategy and knowledge necessary to steward the people You have given us to lead. Thank You for infusing our beings with love that You have for us so that it can be shed abroad to others. Thank You for showing us how to take the resources You have given us to make a place for Your people to meet with You. In Jesus' name. Amen!*

Healthcare Versus Health-CARE

Chapter III

M erriam Webster defines healthcare as "efforts made to maintain or restore physical, mental, or emotional well-being especially by trained and licensed professionals."9 This is a definition that is very familiar to most people. If we were to stand on a corner and randomly select people as they passed by to ask them: 'What is the definition of healthcare?" A considerable number of them would likely respond with words that denote locations, such as a doctor's office, hospital, or clinic. They would likely say health care has to do with "getting well." These thoughts are right in some respect. Healthcare is a system. It is a group of processes with a singular goal. That goal is typically the restoration of well-being.

In the Introduction, we presented a definition of health by Dr. Andrija Štampar. He said, "health is a state of complete physical, mental, and social well-being and not merely the absence of disease or infirmity."[1] The definitions are similar. One might even argue that there is virtually no difference between the two.

Dictionary.com defines CARE as to "feel concern or interest; attach importance to something."[10] It is here that our usage of the word "care" changes.

> "
> Healthcare is a noun, and Health—CARE is a verb."

Healthcare is a person, place, or thing, while Health—CARE is action! It is doing! The **23rd Psalm** is a beautiful depiction of care. It is a Psalm that shows the love of the Father in action.

"The Lord is my shepherd; I shall not want. He maketh me to lie down in green pastures: he leadeth me beside the still waters. He restoreth my soul: he leadeth me in the paths of righteousness for his name's sake. Yea, though I walk through the valley of the shadow of death, I will fear no evil: for thou art with me; thy rod and thy staff they comfort me. Thou preparest a table before me in the presence of mine enemies: thou anointest my head with oil; my cup runneth over. Surely goodness and mercy shall follow me all the days of my life: and I will dwell in the house of the Lord forever" (Psalm 23).

In 1990, through the Office of Disease Prevention and Health Promotion (ODPHP), the United States government introduced its first Healthy People Initiative. It "included the first set of ambitious, measurable 10-year objectives for improving health and well-being nationwide. It focused on decreasing deaths throughout the life span and increasing independence among older adults."[11]

Every 10 years, the objectives are updated. The most current objectives, Healthy People 2030, which was launched in August 2020, emphasize health equity, initiatives that drive social determinants of health, health literacy, and the focus on well-being. The health of the people is a priority. Embracing the fact that health should be a shared goal between the Church and the healthcare system is also a priority. The typical person attends some sort of religious event 1-2 times a week. They do not engage with a healthcare organization this much in most cases. The development of programs that support initiatives such Healthy People are key for the communities that will be affected the most.

Throughout the years, the ODPHP has monitored the success of the initiatives and how well they measure performed through improvements in the health of the people. For instance, in the final report for Healthy People 2000, "some of the major accomplishments include surpassing the target for reducing deaths from coronary heart disease and cancer."[12] Unfortunately, issues of disparity to include accessibility, quality of care, and more remain.

According to the Centers for Disease Control (CDC), "6 of 10 people in the United States have a chronic illness, with 4 of 10 of them have two or more."[3] Chronic illnesses include heart disease, cancer, stroke, and diabetes, to name a few. The risk factors for these conditions are

virtually the same. They are tobacco use, including second smoke, poor nutrition, inactivity, and excessive alcohol use.

Health can be improved by changing some lifestyle habits such as quitting smoking, adopting healthy eating habits, engaging in regular physical activity, knowing familial risk factors, and obtaining regular health screening, to name a few.

As we take this journey, we will discuss health—CARE, the verb, and how the Church can partner with external agencies, its community, and the Word of God to achieve **"Beloved. I wish above all things that thou mayest prosper and be in health, even as thy soul prospereth"** (3 John 2).

Let's pray: *Father, according to Your word in 1 Peter 5:7 Casting all your care upon him; for he careth for you, thank You for caring for us. Thank You for seeing all my issues, concerns, and worries. Please give us a heart for others like Yours so that I can demonstrate the truth of what caring is and not only the noun of healthcare. Show us, Your Church, how to develop a safe place so that others may find the comfort of your care. Give us the revelation of the responsibility of our responsibility as citizens of the Kingdom of God. In Jesus' name. Amen!*

The Prison Church: Mother Consuella B. York-The Lady Preacher

Chapter IV

"The ransom of a man's life are his riches: but the poor heareth not rebuke. The light of the righteous rejoiceth: but the lamp of the wicked shall be put out. Only by pride cometh contention: but with the well advised is wisdom" (Romans 13:8-10).

Ratified in 1791, the first amendment prohibits Congress from interfering in freedom of religion, speech, assembly, or petition. It is here that the principle of "separation of church and state" is derived. Basically, its protective value is to ensure neutrality in the people's pursuit of religious expression. Simply put, there will be no mandated religion in the United States—no government religion. Does this protection include governmental agencies like Departments of Corrections or prisons? Of course, it does. There is no specific religious mandate in the penal system. Because of this freedom, the influence of various religious organizations can be seen. It is here that the story of the little, demure, 5'2 preacher lady from Chicago enters.

As we have established, health is the freedom from "DIS-ease." Certainly, no one would disagree that sin sickness falls under this category. Sin has caused many to fail as lawful, productive members of society. For a group of people to deteriorate morally to such an extent that they would steal, kill, and destroy is a symptom of the lack of health at the core. Jails and prisons overflow with people whose choices, associations, or circumstances caused them to be incarcerated in these subcommunities where they are locked away because the Disease within them has made them a risk—even dangerous—to others. Jesus defined the sources of their sin-sickness. Jesus said in **John 10:10, "The thief comes only to steal and kill and destroy. I came that they may have life and have it abundantly."** To bring life is the role and mission of the Church, a mission that was notably fulfilled in the Prison church set up by Mother Consuella York.

Mother

Consuella Batchelor York was born in Chicago, Illinois, in 1923. Although she entered the world in humble beginnings, her impact on the United States Penal System is still unrivaled more than 25 years after her death.

"Mother" York, also known as the Mother Teresa of the Cook County Jail, began her life's work in the Cook County Department of Corrections (CCDOC) in February of 1952, when an observation day changed her life forever. It also changed the lives of tens of thousands of people that she reached with the soul-saving gospel of Jesus Christ for more than forty-three years.

As a little girl, I remember knowing that Mother York was somebody special. Growing up in her traditional church, the one outside of the jail, I had a front-row seat to watch her life. Being a close family member also gave me insight into the phenomenon known as Mother York. Her genuine love for God's people created a vortex that would sweep you up also if you stood still long enough.

Mother York was born to do great things for the Kingdom of God, "Rev," as my family and those close to her called her, was indeed a force. Through the anointing and the call on her life, she broke down doors of segregation, separatism, and even gender bias. Becoming the first ordained female African American Baptist preacher in Chicago in 1953, Consuella York would later become the jail's first Black chaplain and on to be the Supervisor of Chaplains in 1973. Without question or exception, Mother York took the words of **James 2:1-4** seriously:

"My brethren have not the faith of our Lord Jesus Christ, the Lord of glory, with respect of persons. For if there come unto your assembly a man with a gold ring, in goodly apparel, and there come in also a poor man in vile raiment; And ye have respect to him that weareth the gay clothing, and say unto him, Sit thou here in a good place; and say to the poor, Stand thou there, or sit here under my footstool: Are ye not then partial in yourselves, and are become judges of evil thoughts (James 2:1-4)".

Her love for those who were incarcerated baffled many. They were, in many cases, hardened criminals—murderers, arsonists, thieves, and rapists. But, to her, they were sons. She didn't differentiate between those who attended her regular church or the inmates who attended her Prison church. When questioned about this, she would reply, "I didn't pick the assignment; the Lord picked it for me. After my first visit, I've been a jailbird ever since, serving a life sentence for the Lord."

"Hearken, my beloved brethren, Hath not God chosen the poor of this world rich in faith, and heirs of the kingdom which he hath promised to them that love him? But ye have despised the poor. Do not rich men oppress you, and draw you before the judgment seats? Do not they blaspheme that worthy name by the which ye are called? If ye fulfil the royal law according to the scripture,

> " Thou shalt love thy neighbour as thyself,"

ye do well: But if ye have respect to persons, ye commit sin, and are convinced of the law as transgressors. For whosoever shall keep the whole law, and yet offend in one point, he is guilty of all (James 2:5-13)."

She pastored two congregations, really. The first, I like to say her "real" Church, met every Sunday with her weekly visit to the Cook County Department of Corrections (CCDOC) for service., She also held a Saturday service, where the men were fed the Word of God and chicken dinner—or the Word and "the bird," as they called it. She never came to them empty-handed. Feeding them physically was always next after she fed them spiritually. Her second congregation, organized in 1954, was us. Our "day" would begin at 10am for Sunday School. Here, we learned about the Bible and how to live our lives as Christians. She would arrive "on fire" and ready to go at 1:15pm. She had so much left in her, and we received it all. She completely poured out. Honestly, pastoring two churches, she was ahead of her time. Today, it is common for a pastor to have multiple churches on multiple campuses. In that day, it was highly unusual for a Black Baptist woman to pastor a church at all—certainly, it was a landmark for her to pastor two simultaneously. But again, that was the force of life and love known as Mother York.

Mother York was a stabilizing factor in the lives of many of these men. She insisted that a healthy relationship with God is non-negotiable and priceless. Research studies are full of references to the importance of some sort of religious foundation. The earlier it begins in one's life, the more stabilizing and influential it will be. Consuella York believed and demonstrated that truth at every opportunity.

I asked her only living biological son if he ever felt jealous or slighted because of everybody's love for her. "Never!" he emphatically replied. He then recalled a story when he and his brothers were young and encountered a dog. Immediately she covered them with her own body to protect them from the perceived threat. She never gave any thought to her own safety. Protecting them was her only focus. Shielding people from the danger of sin was her life's mission. There are so many lessons that could be learned from her life. Anyone who met her felt that same sense of intense love and protection in her presence.

Love

The York home was full of love—the love of God and the love of people. Their humble abode could always be found teeming with young people, many of whom came from unstable homes. She literally would give the shirt off her back or the "shoes" off of her own son's feet because that boy "doesn't have a mama like you. she would tell them" Her deep-seated desire to see her sons grow up into respectable members of society colored her entire world. This goal led her to begin her own business that would allow her to be present for them as they navigated the city's dangerous streets. Her printing business gave employment to many from the neighborhood, thereby keeping them off the streets as well.

The love of God she showed was the perfect calling card for God because God IS love. Every week, she, and her wagon with the words "Mother York's goodies" embossed on the side went from cellblock to cellblock, bringing the love of God, His word, toiletries, cakes, and other treats to the men and women incarcerated behind those walls. They also received a corrective word when needed, in addition to a compassionate listening ear. Those men and women received it all, knowing that genuine love was at the heart of what Mother York said and did.

December was a busy time. She and her team of volunteers, many from her church, busied preparing for her annual Christmas feeding of the entire CCDOC. They'd provide a Christmas dinner of turkey and dressing with all the trimmings to every inmate, including the officers and administration. Over 7500 people experienced the love of Christ at the hands of Mother York every year during this annual event.

Two weeks out from her annual Christmas Dinner on December 11, 1995, Mother York went "home for Christmas" when she suffered a major heart attack outside of her beloved church on the Southside of Chicago. The news shook the CCDOC. There was no one like Mother York. She was the only person who could walk the halls during times of unrest and quell the chaos with her mere presence. The inmates were visibly moved by her passing. For many, she was the only mama that they had in their lives. She literally was "the Church." The chaplains whom she had trained flooded the cellblocks to help the inmates cope with this horrible loss, reminding them of her words and her expectations of their behavior. The grief was palpable. In true Mother York fashion, the annual Christmas feeding still happened that year—a testament to her life and love for God and for people.

Her list of accolades could fill this book, but I am sure that she would shrug and say as she always would—"to God be the glory." Honors like the street naming can be found where the church stands to this day, as well as others." The Consuella B. York High School was built on the campus of the CCDOC, and was named in her honor. It is a visible reminder of her commitment to God's people and her knowledge that anyone can rise above their circumstances with God and education. I recall her words,

> " The only difference in us and them is the caught and the un-caught."

Yes, she was a depiction of the Church.

Mother York's love was real and palpable. Small in stature, she was a giant in the Kingdom of God. Her desire for all of mankind was simple: accept Jesus Christ as Savior, then live a life that pleases God. I recall her saying on many occasions, "I wish I could take a hypodermic needle and inject it into people," referring to people loving and living for God. To accept Jesus as Savior and Lord was paramount to pleasing God, and Consuella demonstrated what that looked like in her life.

A heart for the poor and downtrodden is a characteristic that she showed seemingly with ease, but it is one that we are to seek to display as well. How we prove the love of God to others is a hallmark of our Christianity. We are to wear it like we would the jersey of our favorite sports team.

It is not hard to identify a Chicago White Sox or Cubs fan wearing their team regalia. Can't you see them in the stands doing the wave with every home run in a sea of white, black, and silver or white, red, and blue, respectively? You would know that fan if you saw them. What if our love for the seemingly "unlovable" caused us to identify with the very people that Christ died to save—to the point that we became selfless in our pursuit of bringing them to a life of redemption like Mother York? What if our love caused salvation to become a treasured word, rather than a term used in disdain such as "jail house religion?"

Can you imagine a church that hosted programs that not only led people to salvation but to skills that would lead them to be productive members of society? The Bible says in **1 Corinthians 4:15, "For though ye have ten thousand instructors in Christ, yet have ye not many fathers: for in Christ Jesus, I have begotten you through the gospel"** and statistics prove that the impact of fatherless homes can be seen in the U.S. Penal system. The lack of this manly influence has its roots at the core of much of society's woes. The development of male mentoring programs that could provide emotional support and teach skills that assist men in being successful as the head of families is key to repairing this breach in the home.

Having a robust prison ministry like Mother York's may not be possible for every church; however, it is possible for every church to do something. Consider this question as you minister to the spiritual needs of the people in your community: What natural resources and programs are you willing to supply to keep children out of the Penal system before they enter it?

Let's Pray: *Father, thank You for being our good father. Give us Your heart for the fatherless and the wayward as they try to figure out how to navigate this world without stable influences. Teach us how to wear our love as a garment that blesses others and praises You. Help us to be living epistles read of men. In Jesus' name! Amen!*

The Physical Church-The Tent of Meeting

Chapter V

T
he place where the people meet with God is, without doubt, a significant component of the church experience. In **Hebrews 10:24-25**, we are encouraged. **"And let us consider one another to provoke unto love and to good works: Not forsaking the assembling of ourselves together, as the manner of some is but exhorting one another: and so much the more, as ye see the day approaching."** Church buildings around the world range from small "store front" places to large mega churches. The large stately cathedrals with their pipe organs and ornate ceilings and walls are clearly in a class of their own. We all remember the grandeur of the Sistine Chapel.

The Building

While the size of the edifice may interfere with the organization's ability to have outreach opportunities, it does not prevent them. A small one with a commitment to seeing the community prosper can make an impact even though it's not a mega church. Churches of assorted sizes are common in the United States. According to USAChurches.org, "a small church is one with approximately 50 people in attendance on a given weekend, medium with 51-300, large with 301-2000, and mega church would have over 2000."[13] As we discussed in an earlier chapter, it is the mission and vision that has the biggest impact on what and when programs can be developed. It cannot be denied that spatial issues are important. I believe this is one of the reasons that God was so prescriptive with the design of Solomon's temple. Who knows how many outreach programs God was going to inspire there!

The term "tent of meeting" can be found primarily in the Old Testament books of the Bible that make up the Torah. The Tent of Meeting is the place where God met with His people. It was a temporary structure that Moses and the children of Israel brought with them as they traveled to the Promised land. It brings on a different meaning to "Camp Meeting." **"And Moses took the tabernacle, and pitched it without the camp, afar off from the camp, and called it the Tabernacle of the congregation. And it came to pass, that everyone which sought the Lord went out unto the tabernacle of the congregation, which was without the camp"** (Exodus 33:7).

"And it came to pass, as Moses entered into the tabernacle, the cloudy pillar descended, and stood at the door of the tabernacle, and the Lord talked with Moses" (Exodus 33:9).

"And the Lord spake unto Moses face to face, as a man speaketh unto his friend" (Exodus 33:11).

Relationship is a priority for God, as it should be for us. We see here in **Exodus 33:7, 9** that provision had been made to have a place for them to meet with Him. **Verse 9** says, **"the pillar of cloud would come down and stay at the entrance."** Being connected to His people has always been key to God. That is why He sent His only Son to reconcile us back to Him because sin had separated us.

Part A of **Exodus 33:11** says, **"The Lord would speak to Moses face to face, as one speaks to a friend."**

Friendship

I love this verse. It says that Moses spoke with the Lord, face to face as friends! Oh my—that is a relationship goal, for sure. Church attendance has many purposes. One of them is teaching and developing Believers in their walk with God. It shows people how a relationship with the Father is possible to the point that they can also be a "friend of God." Think about that. What an incredible thought it is literally to feel the communication and genuine relationship with Him that is deep and abiding.

Imagine your best friend in the whole wide world. They are the person to whom you tell all your secrets and plans. Sound great, right? It is! But because that person has human flaws, they have the potential to disappoint you. It could even be so significant that you may find it difficult to recover. Oh, but there is a friend that promises never to leave or forsake you. His thoughts towards you are pure, unchanging, and unyielding. **"A man that hath friends must shew himself friendly: and there is a friend that sticketh closer than a brother" (Proverbs 18:24).**

Covenant relationships are foundational in God-ordained structure and operations. Developing healthy, godly relationships should be one of the church's goals. These goals should not merely exist on a mission statement proclamation but should be demonstrated through human interactions as modeled in the sentiment of **Proverbs 18:24.** We need each other.

" Human relationships are in God's design for man"

He said in Genesis it is not good for man to be alone. Of course, He went on to create a woman from Adam. He created her from his rib, which means she was already in him. Wow! Think about that. The answer to the need for companionship and camaraderie is already in you. So, the thought of "I don't need anybody" did not come from God.

Cast that thought down. The Word says in **Proverbs 27:17, "Iron sharpeneth iron; so a man sharpeneth the countenance of his friend."** I am not saying that meaningful relationships cannot be developed outside the church. However, when we realize that the underpinning of true friendship and relationship is love, it is only natural that the church be a representative of it. **Proverbs 17:17** says, **"A friend loveth at all times, and a brother is born for adversity."** This is a true friend. This person has or sees your flaws but loves you away. The verse goes on to say, **"and a brother is born for adversity."** Jesus is our example of true friendship. The House of God is one of the places where we learn about the characteristics of Jesus and God. Knowing God is essential in the life of the Christian. One of the many benefits is having the ability to know the will of the Father. This is gained from having our minds renewed and knowing Him. The ultimate is to know Christ according to **Philippians 3:7-10, "But what things were gain to me, those I counted loss for Christ. Yea doubtless, and I count all things but loss for the excellency of the knowledge of Christ Jesus my Lord: for whom I have suffered the loss of all things, and do count them but dung, that I may win Christ, And be found in him, not having mine own righteousness,** which is of the law, but that which is through the faith of Christ, the righteousness which is of God by faith: That I may know him, and the power of his resurrection, and the fellowship of his sufferings, being made conformable unto his death."

Growth and Development

Impartation is another significant function of the church. According to Merriam-Webster.com, impartation is "the act of imparting something such as knowledge or wisdom."[14] It is granting or communicating something held in store. The Bible puts it this way in **Romans 1:11-12, "For I long to see you, that I may impart unto you some spiritual gift, to the end ye may be established; That is, that I may be comforted together with you by the mutual faith both of you and me."**

The growth and maturity of individuals in the congregation are imperative for developing a healthy corporate church body. Outreach programs are essential to this growth. Being able to host programs that provide value to the community is crucial. Many churches add the original building to account for growth and future planning. It is very common for educational wings, gymnasiums, and larger sanctuaries to be built.

Depending on the community, offering classes such as English as a Second Language (ESL), parenting, and GED classes could provide merit to a church's claim for building up the community from a family, educational and social standpoint. Positioning your community for success spiritually and naturally sets your church apart from others.

Creating a culture that elevates education, enlightenment and enrichment will benefit your church, the individual families, and the community it serves.

> " Education is the vehicle on which hope is driven."

According to Olshansky et al. (2012), "in 2008 white US men and women with 16 years or more of schooling had life expectancies far greater than black Americans with fewer than 12 years of education-14.2 years more for white men than black men, and 10.3 years more for white women than black women."₁5 There are many other examples where the link between education and health is clear. Emphasizing the importance of education demonstrates God's concern for our souls as well as our natural beings.

The development of an educational department is a valuable function regardless of the size of the church or its financial status. Yes, some may have more money to devote to making the programs appear more exciting, but, for adult learners, the concern for how it fits into their lives and what value it brings to them will overshadow the bells and whistles organizers sometimes think are important. For example, a well-planned course that respects attendees' time is more important to the adult learner than one that offers all the bells and whistles but isn't convenient for their work or family schedule.

Knowledge of adult learning principles is essential not only for the development of educational offerings but even for creating other programs, including sermons and curriculum. Valamis.com defined the following principles as key characteristics of adult learners:

1. Adult learners are self-directed and motivated

2. Adult learners use their life experience to facilitate learning

3. Adult learners are goal-driven

4. Adult learners look for relevancy of the information

5. Adult learners are practical

6. Adult learners see and want mentorship

7. Adult learners are open to modern ways of learning

8. Adult learners want to choose how they learn.16

Classes that strengthen both the inner man and the physical man of the congregation should be on the list of programs that are offered. Bible, marriage, and parenting classes are typical offerings that should also be included. Career-focused classes would also be helpful, e.g., Microsoft classes, trades, cooking classes, or senior care classes are other examples. An excellent resource for ideas on strong adult education programs is *50 Ways to Strengthen Adult Education* by Lewis Center for Church Leadership.17 Whenever possible and appropriate, the addition of square footage onto the building may be needed to perform many of the tasks needed to teach the congregants the life skills needed to have healthy lives physically, emotionally, and socially.

The church is not limited to a specific building type with steepled roofs. It is not uncommon to find services being held in recreation centers, event centers, and hotels. As in Moses' day, the tent of meeting, the Church is mobile. We carry the spirit of God with us as we go about our daily lives. 1 **Corinthians 6:19** tells us that our bodies are the temple of the Holy Spirit. We are not our own.

Let's pray: *Father, thank You for allowing us to understand the importance of the physical building as it is here that we meet You. It is here that we learn of You, and it is from here we go out into the world and tell others about You.*

You have given us the mind of Christ so that we may develop programs that honor You and edify Your people. Help us to create a space that represents safety and hope so that Your people will seek You there. As Your Word says, in Proverbs 18:10, "The name of the Lord is a strong tower: the righteous runneth into it and is safe." Thank You for the safety that we find in Your name! In Jesus' name. Amen!

A Shelter in the Time of Storm

Chapter VI

As a child, I always heard phrases like "Jesus is a shelter in the time of storm." As I grew into adulthood, I learned the significant meaning of that truthful phrase! The turmoil of life will give you a greater understanding of the need for shelter— a safe place to retreat into when the storms of life rage. Doubtless, life is full of twists and turns. It is normal. It is to be expected.

Come!

I am reminded of Bible references to a storm and Jesus calming it. Notably, in **Matthew 14:22-33**, we find the account of Jesus walking on water. In this story, Jesus just finished a large preaching "crusade" where thousands of people thronged to hear his words and to see him "heal their sick." The people came from all over. After a while, Jesus performed the miracle of the fishes and loaves by feeding them with two fish and five loaves of bread or, as some have said, "a two-piece fish dinner" when he was moved with compassion over the fact that the people had to be hungry as they had traveled far and stayed for probably hours wanting to receive all that Jesus had to give spiritually.

After sending the disciples away in the boat to the other side, Jesus went up into the mountainside to pray. Later, He came down. The boat was offshore quite a way, but he could see that it was being buffeted by the winds and the waves. Again, showing His concern for the disciples, he walked out on the water towards them. They saw Him and became afraid. Jesus immediately comforted them, telling them not to be afraid and take courage. It was here when Peter asked Jesus if it were really Him to tell him (Peter) to come to meet Him on the water. Jesus replied, "Come!" Peter got out of the boat and walked on the water towards Jesus. Unfortunately, Peter took note of his surroundings and forgot the summons and became afraid and began to sink. He clearly remembered that all he needed to do was to cry out to Jesus, who reached out His hand and caught him saying, "you of little faith, why did you doubt?" Once Peter climbed back into the boat, the winds died down, and the others worshipped Jesus.

As He was with Peter, Jesus is with us during the storms of life. Jesus immediately reached out to rescue Peter. One may criticize Peter for his little faith, but the reality is the storm was raging when he asked Jesus to bid him to come in the first place. He knew that where Jesus was, there was safety. He knew that the ability to weather the storm was present in Jesus. The substance of Peter's faith was his ability to throw his legs over that boat despite everything pointing to reasons not to. As the Church, we must teach people, our disciples, about having the faith to handle the storms of life and having the faith to trust God while walking through the storms. Our confidence is in knowing that His hand is always stretched towards us to provide the answer, the deliverance, and the peace to the winds and waves. Unlike those who would not get out of the boat, Peter now knew what faith in Jesus could accomplish. His faith also blessed the others as they witnessed Peter's miracle. They worshipped Jesus when the storm calmed.

Whether he knew it or not, Peter was a role model. His curiosity, desire for more, and faith in the Master caused the others to see what happens when you "step out," even if for a little bit. The others never walked on water because they never even attempted to get out of the boat. Remember, they thought Jesus was a ghost. Peter was the only one bold enough to ask for proof that it was Jesus walking to them on the water. He knew that if it was really the Master walking on water, He would empower Peter to walk on water, too! People are watching us to see how we handle our storms. Do we cower in a storm, or do we muster up enough faith to even try something that we have never seen done before?

Often, we desire to hide our challenges from people giving the impression that our lives are perfect.

> "
> We have a responsibility to be role models for what happens when we trust God through our storms."

Demonstrating a healthy response to what life looks like is essential for helping people grow up from being "milk drinkers" into people who can take on the meat of the world and thereby have the maturity to handle the various stages of life. We all go through life. I've heard it said this way, we are either in a challenge, on our way out of a challenge, or just finishing a challenge. Life happens to everyone. People will do as we do when we show them the benefits of walking by faith.

We often use the metaphor of a tumultuous sea to describe the chaos that we feel when we are in our pruning and growth season of life. While pruning is necessary for growth, it is not always comfortable.

Jesus said, "I am the true vine, and my Father is the husbandman. Every branch in me that beareth not fruit he taketh away: and every branch that beareth fruit, he purgeth it, that it may bring forth more fruit. Now ye are clean through the word which I have spoken unto you. Abide in me, and I in you. As the branch cannot bear fruit of itself, except it abide in the vine; no more can ye, except ye abide in me. I am the vine, ye are the branches: He that abideth in me, and I in him, the same bringeth forth much fruit: for without me ye can do nothing. If a man abide not in me, he is cast forth as a branch, and is withered; and men gather them, and cast them into the fire, and they are burned. If ye abide in me, and my words abide in you, ye shall ask what ye will, and it shall be done unto you. Herein is my Father glorified, that ye bear much fruit; so shall ye be my disciples" (John 15: 1-8).

Healthy growth and success are directly related to our connection to the VINE. Directly! When the pressures of life come, however, where we find refuge or solace from them makes the difference in how well we survive those pressures. Jesus said to abide in Him, and He will abide in us. Here we see a picture of a healthy relationship. It is a spiritual quid pro quo—something for something.

The "Church" as a Support

All my life, I have heard the Saints say, "you can't beat God giving no matter how hard you try," it is so true. Unfortunately, they were typical speaking of tangible things like money. But God repays us with protections, provision, direction, and more. **Proverbs 19:17** says that when we give to the poor, we lend to the Lord.

God is also the restorer of the brokenhearted and comforts those who mourn. He tells us that His strength is made perfect in our weakness. The question is, where do we obtain our strength when the winds of life blow to the point that you feel that you are about to lose your footing and are about to fall for the last time?

Stress is one of the major causes of mental health/illness issues. Most people can cope and bounce back quickly from its common occurrence. Unfortunately, stress is not a dormant state; it exists on a spectrum. Everyone deals with stress to some degree. The stay-at-home mom can describe her stress as she navigates the emotions about being at home instead of having a traditional job. Working at home may be fulfilling for one person yet stifling for another. The opposite can be true; guilty feelings may surface for someone who is very career-driven and later find themselves tormented by thoughts of leaving things unattended.

Men also experience stress in different ways, which does not minimize the effects and experience of pressure on women. According to Simon A. Rego, Ph.D., speaking on gender differences and the effects of stress, "Men under stress are more likely than women to report having been diagnosed with high blood pressure, type 2 diabetes, and heart disease or heart attack."[18]

The year of the COVID-19 Pandemic will arguably go down in history as one of the most significant stressors ever encountered. Massive shutdowns of businesses, including churches and the need for homeschooling and work from home orders, created unprecedented opportunities for stress and its impact on individuals and families. The fear that blanketed the world was palpable around the globe. The Pandemic was indiscriminate in its devastation related to race, creed, or socioeconomic status. We found ourselves engulfed in a life-changing phenomenon of which the true impact remains to be determined. As of this writing, the ravages of it still grip the world.

The New England Journal of Medicine (NEJM) (2020) reported an increase in intimate partner violence (IPV) during the Pandemic. The

NEJM reports the disproportionate effect on communities of color and other marginalized groups. According to NEJM.org 1:4, women 1:10 men experience physical, emotional, sexual, or psychological abuse from intimate partners. This statistic does not include the impact of domestic violence related to family members, elders, and children.[19]

Church people are not exempt from domestic violence, unfortunately. Providing a safe environment so that people will feel comfortable seeking help is imperative. The Church has a special responsibility related to this very sensitive yet unhealthy element of human life. It is an area where its voice cannot be silent.

As a domestic violence victor—more than a survivor, I know firsthand how people can come to church each week, serve in leadership roles in the ministry, and still suffer in silence because of fear, embarrassment, and even sometimes feeling unworthy of protection. I left home for church on Sundays under a barrage of abuse only to return to its continuation. Yet, I smiled through my tears and served God's people as I earnestly begged Him for deliverance. At the same time, I wanted someone to "see" me. But how could anyone "see" me when my pain was internal?

> "
> A no-tolerance atmosphere for domestic violence must exist in the Church."

Marriage classes, counseling sessions, and sermons are ways this can be accomplished. Children can and must learn the principles of self-respect, self-esteem, and love for others early. The earlier they know, the better. Anger and conflict management are valuable skills. We often think that only adults need them but not true. If that spirit is not arrested early, the playground bully becomes a domestic abuser. Instilling a healthy sense of self-worth undergirded by the Word of God also prepares children and even adults to face and recognize circumstances that come to destroy it.

Protection

The Church serving as a protector of God's people is not new. Do you remember Noah? God gave Him precise instructions about a life-changing event. Let's look at it in **Genesis 6: 14-22, "Make thee an ark of gopher wood; rooms shalt thou make in the ark, and shalt pitch it within and without with pitch. And this is the fashion which thou shalt make it of: The length of the ark shall be three hundred cubits, the breadth of it fifty cubits, and the height of it thirty cubits. A window shalt thou make to the ark, and in a cubit shalt thou finish it above; and the door of the ark shalt thou set in the side thereof; with lower, second, and third stories shalt thou make it. And behold, I, even I, do bring a flood of waters upon the earth, to destroy all flesh, wherein is the breath of life, from under heaven; and everything that is in the earth shall die. But with thee will I establish my covenant; and thou shalt come into the ark, thou, and thy sons, and thy wife, and thy sons' wives with thee. And of every living thing of all flesh, two of every sort shalt thou bring into the ark, to keep them alive with thee; they shall be male and female. Of fowls after their kind, and of cattle after their kind, of every creeping thing of the earth after his kind, two of every sort shall come unto thee, to keep them alive. And take thou unto thee of all food that is eaten, and thou shalt gather it to thee; and it shall be for food for thee, and for them. Thus did Noah; according to all that God commanded him, so did he."**

Noah built the ark to the express dimensions given by God to save his family and the specific animals, clean and unclean. We can learn so much from Noah and the ark related to health—CARE and the Church.

The ark was a shelter or refuge. The ark can be considered as a type of the Church. Therefore, Noah would be a type of church leadership—the Pastor. He was given explicit instructions to keep the animals alive. God told Noah that He (God) would establish His covenant with Noah and his family. As you recall, the world had become increasingly wicked. God even repented that He had made man. But Noah found grace— favor in the eyes of the Lord.

The Church has been given specific instructions as well. Knowing its doctrine is not a denominational statement necessarily, but it is the foundation on which Christ built the Church. Jesus told Peter in **Matthew 16:13-18, "When Jesus came into the coasts of Caesarea Philippi, he asked his disciples, saying, Whom do men say that I the Son of man am? And they said, Some say that thou art John the Baptist: some, Elias; and others, Jeremias, or one of the prophets. He saith unto them, But whom say ye that I am? And Simon Peter answered and said, Thou art the Christ, the Son of the living God. And Jesus answered and said unto him, Blessed art thou, Simon Barjona: for flesh and blood hath not revealed it unto thee, but my Father which is in heaven. And I say also unto thee, That thou art Peter, and upon this rock I will build my church; and the gates of hell shall not prevail against it."**

Everything that Jesus was, and the purpose of His earthly mission is summed up in this verse. Our churches are to be set up to represent Him. He came for the people. He died for the people. So, therefore they should be a place where the people can come to find solace, strength, and substance.

Noah was told to bring the animals in and to keep them alive. Can you imagine what a task that must have been? There were different animals with different needs. One can infer that the animals acted as animals do. There were both predators and prey in the ark. This alone shows the miracle of what God performed at the hand of Noah and his children. The same will be of our churches. Many people of different backgrounds will come to your doors.

> "
> What has God told you about your responsibility to "keep them alive" despite themselves and their self-destructive behaviors?"

The people are looking to the Church to be a place of shelter from their storms. They expect that we have the answers to their questions and suggestions for their dilemmas. Do you have a process for when you notice that "Sister Smith" has bruises on her arms or "Brother Jones" becomes withdrawn and quiet whenever his wife enters the room despite having been in a lively conversation prior? Can you recognize the signs of domestic or child abuse in your congregation, or do you think that is not your concern? Noah had to be vigilant and on guard to keep everyone, including the animals, safe.

When we think of storms and rainy seasons, we think of the noise from the thunder and the messiness from the water. There is also lightning that can be destructive. This is true of the stormy and rainy seasons of life as well. These conditions disturb our peace. They bring a season of "DIS-ease." As a child, were you afraid of rainstorms? As a parent, do your children run to your room when thunder and rain disturbs their peace? Here they come, tattered teddy bear and blanket in tow to your room because they know you will make it all better. They seek you out because they believe that you will restore the peace. You will dispel the "DIS-ease." They find their healthy place with you, even if you are crowded out of bed hanging onto the edge for dear life. They are clueless because, in your presence, they feel better. They feel safe.

It is so with the Church. People will come to find that state of "health." What processes have you put in order to be prepared to care for people in distress?

Food and money are only a few things people seek when they are in chaos personally. Like with our children, when we move over and draw them to our side, they experience the calming love of the Father. The sounds of the rain and the storm become insignificant, and before long, they are sleeping soundly.

God wants us to be that for His people. We are the Place that they will run to. Now, you may be reading this and are not a Pastor, and so you are thinking, "Amen, 'they' need to be ready to support the people of God." Do you remember that you are the Church?

> "
> Do you have an uplifting word in season for the person in the mall who seems down and hopeless, and you get the opportunity to speak into that person's life?"

Do you have an encouraging smile that is like a healing salve for someone who is wounded in their spirit? Can you endeavor to be an ark of safety for someone? Ask God to use you to provide the "shelter" that His people need when the storms of life are raging, and they feel like they are drowning and going down for the last time.

Here are a few examples of resources that you can share as needed:

Suicide Prevention Line: 1-800-273-8255

National Domestic Violence Hotline: 1-800-799-SAFE (7233) or text LOVEIS to 22522

Crisis Hotline: 954-761-1133

Crisis Text Line: Text HOME to 741741

National Parent Hotline: 1-855-427-2736

Child Help National Child Abuse Hotline: 1-800-422-4453

Futures Without Violence: https://www. futureswithoutviolence.org/resources- events/get-help/

Let's pray: *Father, we come to You asking to let us see people as You do. We ask You to grant us understanding and the wisdom to make a difference in the lives of those we encounter. Help us to open our hearts spiritually to release empathy toward them. Equip us to be prepared with a ready word from You and to be prepared to spring into action when their storms of life come. In Jesus' name. Amen!*

Financial Health-The Widow's Mite

Chapter VII

The significance of money was taught early in our home. Unfortunately, financial literacy was not. Financial health is just as important as physical or mental health for the people of God. The lack of this skill leads to many problems for the people.

My family's roots in the church are deep. Our weekly routine began with my grandparents loading up their car with my brother, cousins, and me to take all of us to Sunday School and church. I still wonder how all of us managed to get into that Ford every week. But we piled in, and off we went. I am sure these early days were the imprint of my love for God, His Church, and His people.

Before my grandparents arrived at our house to retrieve my brother, Eric, and me, we had our own rituals. The first one, of course, was making sure that our clothes were immaculate. The second was to get our money for offering. Offering was essential and was one of the most critical steps in our day. Being the eldest, I was considered the responsible one. My brother was the baby. Therefore, things were made simple for him. Every Sunday, we were given fifty cents. Twenty-five cents were for Sunday School. Twenty-five cents were for church.

I was expected to manage my fifty cents regardless of its configuration. I was given more change because I was older and could count the necessary amount for each offering and not lose it. Eric was given two quarters depending on what my parents had, probably what was left from Saturday's trip to the laundromat. Mama felt that two quarters were more manageable for him to keep up with. I, on the other, hand would be given my fifty cents in various ways. Sometimes, I would get a quarter and two dimes and a nickel or two nickels and 4 dimes. Either way, this was a source of significant discomfort for my brother. I remember his Sunday morning crying sessions wailing, "She got more money than me!" After much drama and repeated explanations that we had the same amount of money, we were off to church. Unfortunately, this drama ensued every weekend when we weren't both given two quarters.

My brother's tantrum showed that he understood the significance of money but did not have financial literacy. According to Fernando, "financial literacy is the foundation of your relationship with money, and it is a lifelong journey of learning. The earlier you start, the better off you will be because education is the key to success when it comes to money."[20]

"
A solid financial foundation is essential for the local church."

Jesus demonstrated this concept in this passage when he was questioned about paying taxes.

"**And when they were come to Capernaum, they that received tribute money came to Peter, and said, Doth not your master pay tribute? He saith, yes. And when he was come into the house, Jesus prevented him, saying, what thinkest thou, Simon? of whom do the kings of the** earth take custom or tribute? Of their own children, or of strangers? Peter saith unto him, Of strangers. Jesus saith unto him, then are the children free. Notwithstanding, lest we should offend them, go thou to the sea, and cast an hook, and take up the fish that first cometh up; and when thou hast opened his mouth, thou shalt find a piece of money: that take, and give unto them for me and thee" (Matthew 17:24-27).

Money Answers All Things

Finances are necessary for the church to be able to function well. The building needs repair: utility payments and benevolence for God's people are required. Ministry is a business that involves budgeting and appropriate stewardship of the funds. The above passage demonstrated a miracle for producing money. While God can certainly provide finances this way, it is not likely. The people of God must know their responsibility to supply the house of God with the finances that are needed. The church is run by tithes and offerings.

Giving the tithe, the tenth, has a dual purpose. It benefits the church, but it also helps the giver. **Malachi 3:8-11, "Will a man rob God? Yet ye have robbed me. But ye say, wherein have we robbed thee? In tithes and offerings. Ye are cursed with a curse: for ye have robbed me, even this whole nation. Bring ye all the tithes into the storehouse, that there may be meat in mine house, and prove me now herewith, saith the Lord of hosts, if I will not open you the windows of heaven, and pour you out a blessing, that there shall not be room enough to receive it. And I will rebuke the devourer for your sakes, and he shall not destroy the fruits of your ground; neither shall your vine cast her fruit before the time in the field, saith the Lord of hosts."**

Let's talk about the benefit to the church first. When the people tithe faithfully, the Bible says that storehouses are supplied with meat. It is provided with the sustenance that the Church needs to function. This even means paper, pens, etc. The Bible also speaks of the responsibility to care for the widow and the orphan.

"Pure religion and undefiled before God and the Father is this, To visit the fatherless and widows in their affliction, and to keep himself unspotted from the world" (James 1:27).

"He doth execute the judgment of the fatherless and widow, and loveth the stranger, in giving him food and raiment" (Deuteronomy 10:18).

"If a brother or sister be naked, and destitute of daily food, And one of you say unto them, Depart in peace, be ye warmed and filled; notwithstanding ye give them not those things which are needful to the body; what doth it profit" (James 2:15-16)?

We benefit when we tithe. Helping the church care for the widow, the orphan, and the less fortunate is one of the benefits. God said, "prove me," and see if HE won't open the windows of heaven and pour YOU out a blessing that you won't have room enough to receive. There is a blessing for the tither that is in abundance. The Father says that "He" would pour. The Bible says He would take on the responsibility to see that you are blessed immeasurably, IMMEASURABLY. He then goes on to say that He would rebuke the devourer for you. It is here that you can call God into remembrance of His word. I have had to more than once say, "I'm a tither," so the devourer is rebuked for my sake when something would break or was even stolen. The tithe is the ultimate insurance policy because it establishes honor for God as your priority. And God said He will honor those who honor Him! **(1 Samuel 2:30).**

Setting a culture amongst one's congregation related to education and maintaining employee or entrepreneurship is essential. This can be done by teaching and impartation. The size of the congregation does not determine whether the church is financially stable. The people's commitment to the financial health of their church is what matters.

"Then they that gladly received his word were baptized: and the same day there were added unto them about three thousand souls. And they continued steadfastly in the apostles' doctrine and fellowship, and in breaking of bread, and in prayers. And fear came upon every soul: and many wonders and signs were done by the apostles. And all that believed were together, and had all things common; And sold their possessions and goods, and parted them to all men, as every man had need" (Acts 2:41-45).

A healthy body of Believers is not just made up of tithers and givers. They are also forward thinkers to ensure that the house of God has everything that it needs. Some Churches host financial classes on budgeting, credit repair, and debt freedom. All of these not only benefit the individuals but also benefit the church. We see in Haggai that God has a strong expectation for His people to care for His house.

"Thus saith the Lord of hosts; Consider your ways. Go up to the mountain, and bring wood, and build the house, and I will take pleasure in it, and I will be glorified, saith the Lord. Ye looked for much, and, lo it came to little; and when ye brought it home, I did blow upon it. Why? saith the Lord of hosts. Because of mine house that is waste, and ye run every man unto his own house" (Haggai 1:7-9).

Caring for the poor, caring for widows and orphans takes money. Fundraisers and fried chicken dinner sales have become one of the ways that churches supplement their finances. Still, the Bible is clear on how the work of the church is to be financed.

> " When we give to the work of the Lord, we will always be blessed."

Setting this expectation positions the people of God to be blessed as they bless the house of God.

"And the word of the Lord came to Solomon, saying, Concerning this house which thou art in building, if thou wilt walk in my statutes, and execute my judgments, and keep all my commandments to walk in them; then will I perform my word with thee, which I spake unto David thy father: And I will dwell among the children of Israel, and will not forsake my people Israel" (1 Kings 6:11-13).

Let's pray: *Father, we thank you for Your revelation on the importance of supporting the house of God. We thank You for showing us in Your Word that we give to it; You reward us. In Jesus' name. Amen*

The Power of the Praying Church

Chapter VIII

Prayer is the bedrock of the Church. The congregation that builds its foundation on prayer is one whose people will see and experience the miraculous provisions of God regularly. Consistent prayer and fasting corporately set a church apart from its peers by leaps and bounds. It is a power-filled, spirit-led church. It is here that you can see an outworking of the quote: "Prayer is the key, and faith unlocks the door."

This function of the church should not be relegated to the ministerial staff only. Understanding how to pray or "how to get a prayer through" is something that not only should be demonstrated but can be taught. Persistence in prayer is a skill. It is one that every Believer should have in their toolbox for Christian living.

Answered prayer and signs and wonders are guaranteed when we go to Him in faith, believing, without doubt. The Bible tells us the angels

> "Access to God through prayer using His Word is a sure way to experience the Kingdom come to earth as it is in heaven."

harken to the Word of God. They get busy when we pray it boldly with expectation **(Psalm 103:20).**

Teaching Believers to use the Word of God with the confessions of their hearts is a fundamental responsibility of the Church. Learning how to speak life into the various circumstances of life is imperative. Healing and wholeness ultimately are given to us by God. Through His sovereignty, He chooses how to heal. But He has given us His Word to use a weapon to destroy the kingdom of darkness. Communication with God in prayer is one of the strongest weapons we have. Knowing the power of our words is critical. However, He also uses modern medicine. There is a great power that comes to bear when we pray the Word of God. Declaring and decreeing God's Word over our situations and lives creates a level of anticipation that brings results.

Modern medicine is another way God has given us to bring health to His people. The Word of God is full of references to doctors and medicine. Luke was a physician. He was one of Paul's co-workers in ministry. Being a Believer in Jesus Christ does not preclude Christians from engaging with the medical community. In fact, they make good partnerships. Notice I used the word partnership. The medical community is simply one of the tools God uses. They have similar goals and missions as it relates to the health of the community.

Healing is manifested in many ways according to our faith. Without a doubt, the power of life and death is in our mouths. **Proverbs 18:21 says, "Death and life are in the power of the tongue: and they that love it shall eat the fruit thereof."**

Sister Mary

Mary was an amazing woman of God. She was filled with God's spirit and compassion for His people. Her leadership could be felt and seen throughout the organization. Unfortunately, Mary was given a cancer diagnosis that she ignored. She continued to ignore the diagnosis as she continued to stand in what she thought was faith until years later, the results of not following the medical advice turned terminal. She succumbed to the disease, leaving her family and the Kingdom with unfinished assignments and possibly others confused.

Many questions can be asked about this example.

1. Did she seek God for the direction to take regarding the diagnosis?
2. What really kept her from following the doctor's advice? Was it fear?
3. Did she surround herself with the prayers and support of other like-minded Believers who could cover in prayer, believing God for her healing?

I am not judging Mary's decision or her faith. Chapter 9 answers those questions. They are items for consideration when you are facing a situation like hers. There is one thing for sure, a soldier left the earth too soon. As people of God, we must genuinely stand on faith and not merely "sticking our heads in the sand." **"Now faith is the substance of things hoped for, the evidence of things not seen" (Hebrews 11:1).**

If you have children, you will understand this analogy. Father God is a good father who gives excellent gifts to His children. As humans, we give gifts to our children as well. Have you ever promised your children something special? How often did they ask you about it before they received it? They continually asked, inquired after, reminded you about it. They did it repeatedly until you finally presented them with the long-awaited promise. As irritating as it was, they were right! Matthew 7:7 says, **"Ask, and it shall be given you; seek, and ye shall find; knock, and it shall be opened unto you."** Another translation says, ask and keep on asking, seek and keep on seeking and knock and keep on knocking. Keep it up. The powerhouse church has mastered the art of persistent prayer and teaches its members how to master it. We can learn a lot about prayer from observing our children's tenacity and perseverance in making their requests known.

God's Word is full of promises—full! He tells us in 2 Corinthians 1:20, "For all the promises of God in him are yea, and in him Amen, unto the glory of God by us." He goes further to say in Isaiah 43:26, "Put me in remembrance: let us plead together: declare thou, that thou mayest be justified."

Speak it!

"Then said the Lord unto me, Thou hast well seen: for I will hasten my word to perform it." He wants His promises to be manifested in our lives. When we ask and keep on asking, it doesn't "get on his nerves," but to the contrary, it demonstrates our faith in the fact that He will reward us if we diligently seek Him. God sees it as we are standing on what He has said. Praying the scriptures or giving God His Word back happens when we take it and emerge ourselves into its very essence.

> "
> This requires taking the scripture and seeing it literally as being alive and active."

Teaching the skill of personalizing it will show how true that statement is.

Decreeing and declaring the scripture is another skill that can be taught. Teach people how to take the Word of God and wield it as the two-edged sword that it is. Confessing it also yields great reward. Please refer to the back of this book and review Appendices A-C as examples of decrees, declarations, as well as confessions you can personalize and incorporate into your own life. Can you imagine the exploits you can do for the Kingdom once you realize that God's Word is full of promises waiting to be taken and used in life?

The congregation taught the significance that this power will give God the greatest honor by believing His Word. The Church that understands this will be unstoppable, prosperous, and healthy.

Let's Pray: *Father, as Jesus taught the disciples to pray, please teach us the importance of prayer. Help us to realize that it is communication with You. Help us to know that You have the answer to all our questions, the peace to lift us out of all chaos, and to provide the joy that gives us strength when we are weak. In Jesus' name! Amen!*

Mental Illness: Dispelling the Stigma

Chapter IX

Mental health is the overall feeling of physical, emotional, and social well-being. While often used interchangeably with mental illness, it is not the same. The American Psychiatric Association says, "Mental illnesses are health conditions involving significant changes in thinking, emotion, or behavior (or a combination of these)."[21]

The average person considers mental illness to be a condition such as schizophrenia or bipolar disorder. However, it is more than these types of illnesses. According to the National Institute of Mental Health (NIMH), one in five adults in the United States lives with a mental illness.[22] Mental illness ranges from depressions to those that debilitate and affect the person's abilities in one or more major life activities. Insomnia, excessive anxiety, and addiction/substance abuse are also examples. Children also suffer from varying degrees of mental illness. Diseases such as personality disorders, eating disorders, and even autism spectrum disorder can be found in children.

Hollywood has painted a picture of what mental illness looks like, which is often far from reality. Movies such as *One Flew Over the Cuckoo's Nest*, circa 1975, depict the inside of a psych ward that is not entirely factual. While I suppose it made for good entertainment, it did not help with the dismissal of the stereotypes that still stigmatize those who suffer from these disorders today. Jack Nicholson's character and Nurse Ratchet's engagement in an emotional and physical interactive war against wills made for exciting cinematography. Yet, it gave an unrealistic view of what those who seek medical/psychological assistance experience in today's world. Contrary to the idea of the movie, most people with a mental illness don't go around talking to themselves or rocking back and forth. Instead, most are contributing members of society.

I recall an incident while serving as the Infection Prevention (IP) manager for a former employer. While performing rounds on one of the psych units, I had a memorable interaction with one of the patients. Being focused on my assignment, I found myself in the crosshairs of one of the residents on the unit. This was not just any hospital unit and should not have been treated as such.

My partner and I were walking around assessing for environmental, infectious risks. After all, I was in my element. Those risks could not hide from me! I was there to seek them out and ensure that they were taken care of so that "my" patients were safe. Armed with one of the most valuable tools that an IP could have, a camera, my colleague and I toured the unit looking top to bottom for things that needed to be corrected. Infection prevention was necessary even on the psych unit.

Unbeknownst to me, while I was looking for potential risks to the patients in the environment, I was being watched by one of them. I snapped a couple of pictures of things that needed to be addressed but, of course, not of the patients. I knew better than that! I must have taken one shot too many when my partner and I entered the unit's laundry room. Suddenly, we heard screaming from across the dayroom, "Hey! You can't do that!" the gentleman yelled. Still clueless, I snapped a couple more pictures in the laundry room. "What?" I replied, stepping out of the laundry room to see who was talking to me. My colleague was uneasy from the beginning of rounds because most people did not like going there. In response to the commotion, she closed the door, securing herself inside, leaving me outside the laundry room, trying to find out what the problem was. I wasn't concerned about my safety. I wanted to know what he was talking about. On the other side of the dayroom was another patient who was oblivious to what was going on. The angry patient continued to yell, "You can't do that! I know my rights!"

I recall trying in vain to explain that I wasn't taking a picture of him as he continued to tell me about "his rights." He never advanced towards me, but the anger in his voice continued to grow in intensity. The charge nurse finally heard the commotion. She obviously wasn't concerned about me or my camera until now.

She immediately walked over using verbal de-escalation techniques to calm the patient that I had infuriated. He yelled, "She can't be taking pictures! I know my rights." The nurse replied to him, "Oh, that's Phyllis—she's over Infection Prevention and is here to make sure that everything is safe for you."

"Then she should know better," he responded, beginning to calm down.

He was utterly unimpressed with my title. On the other hand, I was internally bristling as my own trigger for being called "she" was being activated. I am still not sure why that bothers me. But as the manager of Infection Prevention, I couldn't start acting like another out-of-control "psych patient" on the unit just because he hit one of my own triggers. So, I halted my own internal issue as I tried to explain what I was doing and that I had not taken his picture. He totally ignored and dismissed me and kept speaking with the nurse. Clearly, he was convinced that I was an idiot who didn't know better and, therefore, didn't merit any more of his time.

As the nurse kept quieting the patient, I quietly went to the laundry room to retrieve my partner, who had barricaded herself behind the door. "Let's go," I said. Our work for the unit was done—at least for that day. As we left the unit, I could see the formerly irate patient eyeing me with a smirk that said, "You should have known better...I know my rights!"

Once my colleague and I were safely on the other side of the locked doors and out of earshot, we erupted into uncontrollable laughter. She had totally abandoned me, and the fact is, I "should have known better!" She had left me without an advocate.

Although mentally ill, that man was very self-aware and was his own advocate. He knew his rights and had no problem standing up for them. As the Church, we are responsible for advocating for those who cannot. Our congregations are full of people who need someone to help and support them, a loose definition of the word "advocate."

The Advocate

Jesus, too, encountered a man who needed an advocate.

> "
> Unlike me, Jesus is the ultimate Advocate and continues to be so today for us all. "

The story of Jesus and the man from Gadara was very different from mine and ended much better. Here we find Jesus and his disciples coming off an incident when He had just calmed the storm from which his disciples were afraid. Jesus asked them why they were worried. Didn't they have faith? Our story takes us from Jesus calming tumultuous sea to a man with an explosive spirit in **Mark 5:1-20:**

"And they came over unto the other side of the sea, into the country of the Gadarenes. And when he was come out of the ship, immediately there met him out of the tombs a man with an unclean spirit, Who had his dwelling among the tombs; and no man could bind him, no, not with chains: Because that he had been often bound with fetters and chains, and the chains had been plucked asunder by him, and the fetters broken in pieces: neither could any man tame him. And always, night and day, he was in the mountains, and in the tombs, crying, and cutting himself with stones. But when he saw Jesus afar off, he ran and worshipped him, And cried with a loud voice, and said, What have I to do with thee, Jesus, thou Son of the most high God? I adjure thee by God, that thou torment me not. For he said unto him, Come out of the man, thou unclean spirit. And he asked him, What is thy name? And he answered, saying, My name is Legion: for we are many. And he besought him much that he would not send them away out of the country. Now there was there nigh unto the mountains a great herd of swine feeding. And all the devils besought him, saying, Send us into the swine, that we may enter into them. And forthwith Jesus gave them leave. And the unclean spirits went out and entered into the swine: and the herd ran violently down a steep place into the sea, (they were about two thousand;) and were choked in the sea. And they that fed the swine fled, and told it in the city, and in the country. And they went out to see what it was that was done. And they come to Jesus, and see him that was possessed with the devil, and had the legion, sitting, and clothed, and in his right mind: and they were afraid. And they that saw it told them how it befell to him that was possessed with the devil, and also concerning the swine. And they began to pray him to depart out of their coasts. And when he was come into the ship, he that had been possessed with the devil prayed him that he might be with him. Howbeit Jesus suffered him not, but saith unto him, Go home to thy friends, and tell them how great things the Lord hath done for thee, and hath had compassion on thee. And he departed and began to publish in Decapolis how great things Jesus had done for him: and all men did marvel."

This is a very familiar story from the Bible. It presents the circumstances of the man from the Gadara who had a mental illness. He was also possessed by evil spirits. Despite the prevalent belief, mental illness is not to be confused with possession of evil spirits. However, it is possible that it can co-exist just like a person can have diabetes and be blind. These are two different medical conditions that can co-exist in one individual. The way Jesus handled this tormented man from Gadara is a blueprint for us today.

The stigma and prejudice experienced by the man unfortunately still exists today. Many similarities can be drawn from how he was viewed then and how mentally ill people are generally viewed today. First, he was identified as his condition. He is often called the Madman of Gadara or the Gadarene Demoniac. Have you ever noticed this happen? People are often identified by their condition. This pronouncement continues to validate the power that the condition has versus the delivering power of Jesus Christ. I have seen people called by an unfavorable condition in their body or circumstance and have always wondered: *How does that defining label make them feel?*

Names that negatively refer to a person's physical stature, skin color, birthmarks, and body size can engender feelings of inadequacy and inferiority. Such negativity can at some point cause people to internalize the identifying label and begin to even refer to themselves by these names, fortifying its harmful effects and giving rise to other negative expressions.

The people of the Gadara community were unable to deal with this man's behavior despite their attempts to do so.

> "What preparations should you make to care for people with various struggles?"

Is there an inherent responsibility that it holds? I find it interesting that the scripture says that he cried out "night and day in the tombs and in the hills." This man knew that what was going on in him was not right. He did not like what he had become. His behavior was not simply an irritant to others, but it was a cry for help. Who would love living among the dead things—no one would?

But deep inside, his spirit recognized his need for Salvation. He ran to Jesus. Some interpretations say he worshipped Jesus. Even still, the evil spirits oppressing him recognized Jesus and begged Him not to send them out of the man. They knew that Salvation power was present even before Jesus ever uttered a word. Jesus proceeded to command it to come out of the man, asking it, "what is your name?" The spirit replied, "legion because we are many." Again, we see the significance of a name.

People are suffering many things. Some are professionally diagnosed, and others are not. They come to us seeking help. We must be prepared to respond—not just with programs but with the power of God. The spirit crying out through that man begged Jesus not to send the legion into the area but into a herd of nearby pigs. Again, it recognized the Power that was present in Jesus. Jesus sent them into the pigs, which immediately ran down the hill and drowned themselves. Every spirit must submit to the command of Jesus, and He has given us the same power by the authority of His Name. We can provide relief to those who are being tormented mentally and physically.

Jesus said in **John 14:12, "Verily, verily, I say unto you, He that believeth on me, the works that I do shall he do also; and greater works than these shall he do; because I go unto my Father."** You may be thinking as you read this, *Phyllis, are you saying that I can speak in the Name of Jesus, and evil spirits will obey me?* I am absolutely saying that because Jesus said it! **(Matthew 18:18; John 14:13; Luke 10:19).**

This story is glorious because the man was set free, but it gets better! The same townspeople who witnessed this man's torment saw the man "clothed and in his right mind" because of Jesus! These were the same people who had seen him running around naked and hurting himself. They had been afraid of him. But now there, he was completely delivered, clothed, and sitting with Jesus. I find it interesting that this scared them also.

The now delivered man wanted to follow Jesus, but Jesus told him to go instead back to his home and tell others about what God had done for him. This man, who was once naked and cutting himself in the tombs amongst the dead things, became an evangelist, testifying of the power of deliverance at the hands of Jesus! What could happen if the Church walked in the authority that Christ died to give us? What could happen if we walked into our dead communities and called out the legions from among the people. What if we embodied the same power that Jesus said we would display if we only believed? Did he say more extraordinary things would be accomplished through the power of His Name? Your church might be full of people who have mental issues that need deliverance. What a glorious problem! That problem becomes the platform for God's power to be displayed! Wouldn't it be wonderful to be known as the place where people can get delivered and set free and then sent out as witnesses to the power of God that is at work in your church!

Being equipped with the resources necessary to aid and assist all of God's children is essential. Here are some basic things you can do to prepare to minister in this area.

1. Know your limitations even if you are a licensed professional counselor.
2. Maintain a list of resources for referral needs.
   • *Mental Health—A Guide for Faith Leaders*[23]
   • *Top 10 Resources for Mental Health Ministry*[24]
   • *Health and Wholeness—Resources for Mental Health Ministries*[25]
3. Be present with all members, including those with a mental illness. Ensure that your Benevolence Committee includes them. Treat them like any other sick member of your church.
4. Destigmatize it in your congregation. Don't allow words like "crazy" to be used in regular speech.
5. Organize a support group that is run by a Nurse Practitioner or Mental Health Professional
   • Alcoholics Anonymous class
   • Narcotics Anonymous class
   • Stress Management class
   • Conflict Management class

To try to provide resources and offer information in addition to prayer and Scriptural instruction is valuable. In doing this, you will demonstrate the practical application of spiritual help and professional instruction that will combine to change lives. This will enable it to make a significant and lasting difference in your community.

Let's pray: *Father, according to John 14:12, we believe in Jesus and the works that He performed, and because of that, we can do the works He performed and greater. Please help us stand firmly on Your Word, knowing that people need us to walk in the authority He gave us. In Jesus' name. Amen!*

Embracing the Church's Role

Chapter X

We have discussed various ways the Church shares the responsibility for the health of its community. The early Church demonstrated this belief by "having all things common" **(Acts 2:44, 45)**. They knew the importance of community. Using modern-day terminology, one could say that they embodied the "golden rule"—Do unto others as you would have them do unto you.

The 21st-century church can teach and demonstrate Jesus's love through His ministry on earth. Unfortunately, this takes some mindset shifting in many cases. We live in a world that has become colder and more selfish.

God is love, and He demonstrated that love for us by giving His only son to die for our sins and woes, all while we were enemies to Him **(Romans 5:8,10)**. One of the significant roles that we play is to model that love as well.

> "Teaching others to live God-honoring, healthy lives is a way to embrace this role."

The concept of "all things in common" is needed now more than ever in the world that we live in. The moral compass has veered far from God's intent for humanity and the Kingdom. We are separated by race, ethnicity, socioeconomic status, and even religion. Yes, we are far from the intent of **Acts 2:44.**

The Church That Serves

"Charity suffered long and is kind; charity envieth not; charity vaunteth, not itself, is not puffed up, doth not behave itself unseemly, seeketh not her own, is not easily provoked, thinketh no evil; rejoiceth not in iniquity, but rejoiceth in the truth; beareth all things, believeth all things, hopeth all things, endureth all things. Charity never faileth: but whether there be prophecies, they shall fail; whether there be tongues, they shall cease; whether there be knowledge, it shall vanish away" (1 Corinthians 13:4-8).

To be a physically, emotionally, and financially healthy church, we must also become spiritually mature. These characteristics are important as we grow God's people. Love underpins everything that we do as the body of Christ.

The attribute of being a loving church is imperative as it embraces the fact that it has a Kingdom responsibility to focus on the health of the people of God. A loving church is a giving church, and a giving church is a healthy church. Now, hold on before you think that by giving, we are only talking about finances. The truth is financial giving is a small part. Often hosting an event such as a class taught by someone in your church will have little overhead, especially when the people have the heart to serve. So, maybe I should say it this way, a loving church is a serving church, and a serving church is a healthy church. Let's look at **Ephesians 3:14-21.**

"For this cause I bow my knees unto the Father of our Lord Jesus Christ, Of whom the whole family in heaven and earth is named, That he would grant you, according to the riches of his glory, to be strengthened with might by his Spirit in the inner man; That Christ may dwell in your hearts by faith; that ye, being rooted and grounded in love, May be able to comprehend with all saints what is the breadth, and length, and depth, and height; And to know the love of Christ, which passeth knowledge, that ye might be filled with all the fulness of God. Now unto him that is able to do exceeding abundantly above all that we ask or think, according to the power that worketh in us, Unto him be glory in the church by Christ Jesus throughout all ages, world without end. Amen."

The Bible says that Jesus went about doing good (Acts 10:38). He sought opportunities to serve. Jesus led by serving those who were downtrodden and oppressed by life and even satanic forces. This posture encouraged others to serve as well.

> "
> What opportunities to serve your community has your church sought out?"

Are you located in a neighborhood with a sizeable elderly population where a *Meals-on-Wheels* site would be beneficial? What about starting an after-school program for the children in the neighborhood whose parents work and are home alone? The church could help with tutoring and homework and keep the children safe and off the streets.

Have you ever thought about what attracts laborers to your vineyard? The Word tells us that the fields are white, the harvest is ready, but there is a lack of workers. People are attracted to churches that are active and alive. A church that is busy in the community and is a beacon of light and hope is one where people seek to have an opportunity to help others. People are also attracted to the benevolence of churches. It is not uncommon for people who once were on the receiving side to become the best members and givers. Can you imagine your church bustling with activity during the week as well as on weekends? This sounds like an innovative, spirit-led church that exemplifies being the "hand and feet" of Jesus. **"As we have, therefore, opportunity, let us do good unto all men, especially unto them who are of the household of faith" (Galatians 6:10).**

Caring for the mind, body, and spirit of the citizens of the Kingdom falls within the job description of the Church. Loving, giving, and serving are primary in the description.

Let's Pray: *Father, Your Word instructs us to ask You when we find ourselves confused or lacking wisdom. It is our desire to be examples of You on the earth. Like You have given us pastors after Your own heart, please infuse us with those same characteristics that will make us value our responsibility to Your Church. Help us be Your hands and feet as Your Kingdom on earth represents that which is in heaven. In Jesus' name! Amen!*

Designing a Rapha Health Ministry

Chapter XI

When I was a child, I remember the church having a nurses' board. This group of women provided care to the pastor during Worship Services. They typically sat behind the pastor with pristine white uniforms with nurses' caps. One did not even have to be a nurse to serve in this capacity. She would provide water or other drinks to the pastor to keep them hydrated and handkerchiefs to dry up perspiration. From my vantage point, these individuals were commissioned to only care for the pastor and maybe others in the pulpit.

As time has gone on, the role of the church nurse has seemed to diminish into one of an armorbearer, someone who serves the pastor or other members of the clergy in a variety of ways which includes the tasks of the former "nurse" but also includes tasks like that of a security detail. Clearly, this is not a health ministry.

> " A health ministry is a department in a church whose major focus is the health and wellness of the congregation. "

Many years ago, I developed a health ministry for my church. It was called the Rapha Ministry after Jehovah Rapha—the God that heals! This group performed many tasks related to the health and wellness of the congregation, from immediate assistance during health emergencies to organizing and directing health-related events. Let us look at an outline for developing one for your organization. A well-structured health ministry is imperative for several reasons. The well-trained team minimizes mistakes and limit chances for litigation for your church. Yes, I said litigation. Church people bring lawsuits as well.

I. Obtain the sanction and authority from the Senior Pastoral leader

   a. This is essential towards getting the buy-in from the rest of the leaders and the congregants. Examples of buy-in: Cardiovascular Health Awareness Day-someone gives a heart health-related sermon, and the health ministry does blood pressure screenings after church.

   b. Find a name for the ministry. This validates the ministry and legitimizes it. Examples of names: Rapha Ministry, Healing & Wholeness Ministry, the Balm in Gilead Committee

   c. Find a scripture reference on which the ministry will stand.

II. Appoint someone to serve as the ministry servant leader. Preferably, this individual should be a nurse. If not, someone who works in healthcare will work out.

   a. Make a call for volunteers

   b. Develop job descriptions for the volunteer team

   c. Collect and keep current copies of licensure for staff with healthcare licenses.

d. Develop a set of policies and procedures that govern the standard operating procedures (SOP) of the ministry related to the various activities of the ministry, e.g., emergency management, outreach, inhouse ministries — the nursery, etc.

e. Develop a supply list, e.g., BP cuff, bandages, etc.

f. Develop a schedule for the team of who is on duty and for which service

g. Will the ministry be uniformed? (I recommend this. This allows for quick identification of the ministry team in the event of an emergency)

h. Set a meeting and training schedule for the team.

i. Know who holds a CPR certification and when it expires. (I recommend that your nursery staff have CPR training as well as rescue training. Minutes are precious. They should know how to begin to respond before your health ministry staff arrives)

j. Will the church have an Automated External Defibrillator AED? Who will be trained to use it?

III. Determine the goals and mission of the ministry. Will your health ministry only respond to emergencies? (I hope not. There is so much fun to be had!) How many health-related events will you host a year?

IV. Determine if the ministry will be allotted an independent budget or if it will be required to seek approvals for every need. Either way is acceptable. However, it is essential to know because some minor expenditures will need to be made. The size of the church will determine what that budget should look like.

Let's pray: *Father, please give us insight as we yield to the mind of Christ in organizing a health ministry that glorifies You and edifies Your people. Give us witty inventions and creative ideas in our sleep that will cause this ministry to remove burdens and destroy yokes. In Jesus' name. Amen!*

Divine Connections

Chapter XII

We have discussed the healthy church and the CARE of its people.

" Empowerment, impartation, and organization are the pillars of a healthy congregation. "

Fortunately, you do not have to re-invent the wheel. Partnership is key. It is critical to know who and what your resources are in your church. Is there someone who can donate a wheelchair to the ministry (an essential piece of equipment)? Do you have an educator who will be happy to help with curriculum development? Is someone handy and can build a ramp if needed? Assessing the state of your house will save you lots of money upfront. You could have a significant portion of what you need already there. There will be people who want to be of assistance but have no medical training. Allowing someone to help with administrative duties is a great way to divide all the responsibilities and not overwhelm one person.

There are many community resources that you can take advantage of. Search your locale for organizations such as Congregational or Parish Nursing. These groups can support your organization where you may lack it internally.

Develop a resource guide for your church. You must have all the resources for your health ministry in one place at your fingertips. You need to know who to call for elder care questions or mental health concerns, for example. Gather all these contacts and place them with the SOPs. It is also vital that you touch bases with the organization to have a cursory relationship. Staying in touch with them will also keep your church top of mind when they get resources. Non-profits like this are often beneficiaries of items that would bless your church greatly. Knowing the contact information for the company that supplies transportation for the elderly is also a great asset.

Knowing what conditions your congregants have is important as you plan educational offerings for your church. You may not want to require people to report every ache and pain to the church office but having a way to "be present" in the lives of your members is very important. This is how you exhibit health—CARE. There is a way to gather this information without being intrusive. As you can imagine, it is critical to know if someone in your congregation has diabetes. Being armed with this information is essential so that your health ministry will learn how to respond without wasting valuable time, for example. Once people realize that the church focuses on health, they will often volunteer this information to the appropriate people. Maintaining privacy and confidentiality must be an utmost priority.

Providing consistent education on various health-related topics either across the pulpit or in the church newsletter will quickly drive a transformational view of health in your church. These focuses have already been put together; all you will need is to make the information fit your church culture by determining how they learn and retain information best.

Every year in February is American Heart Month, and there is a National Wear Red Day. Making a church-wide celebration around observations like this will demonstrate your commitment to the church's health. October is Domestic Violence Awareness Month. Not ignoring this significant month shows your congregation that this topic is a high priority, and that domestic violence is not tolerated.

Having a church that values health is the beginning of a church that will be long-standing. We see the theme running throughout the Bible. Health and wholeness were God's ideas. Jesus was wounded for our sins and by His stripes were and are healed. A healthy church honors the sacrifice of the One who said: "I come that you might have life."

Combining solid health care and our covenant cure—Jesus Christ—let's go into our communities being the Church. We are to fulfill the mandate to bring life and that more abundantly... especially to "the least of these."

The thief cometh not, but for to steal, and to kill, and to destroy: I am come that they might have life, and that they might have it more abundantly (John 10:10).

Let's Pray: *Father, You demonstrated the importance of human connections when You said it is not good for man to be alone. You have shown us that we are better together. Lead us to godly partnerships that further Your mission for us as we seek to carry it out Your way and not ours. Help us to be good partners in return. In Jesus' name. Amen!*

Appendix A

Scriptures To Release Life and Health into Your Spirit, Soul, and Body

My son, pay attention to what I say; turn your ear to my words. Do not let them out of your sight, keep them within your heart; for they are life to those who find them and health to one's whole body. Above all else, guard your heart, for everything you do flows from it (Proverbs 4:20-23 NIV).

Beloved, I pray that you may prosper in all things and be in health, just as your soul prospers (3 John 2 NKJV).

God's words are spirit and life (*see* **John 6:63**). When you choose to believe and release words and affirmations that agree with what God says about you, those confessions will produce health and wholeness in every area of your life. Even angelic assistance will respond to His words voiced through your confessions.

With corresponding affirmations and confessions, these scriptures will release life, strength, and wholeness into you and your situations as you speak to them. Read through them and allow the words to speak to you.

"For verily I say unto you, That whosoever shall say unto this mountain, Be thou removed, and be thou cast into the sea; and shall not doubt in his heart, but shall believe that those things which he saith shall come to pass; he shall have whatsoever he saith. Therefore I say unto you, What things soever ye desire, when ye pray, believe that ye receive them, and ye shall have them" (Mark 11:23-24).

Father, according to Your Word in **Mark 11:23-24**, I will use my mouth to say what your Word has said about every circumstance that affects me. I will not doubt but believe only. I will ask, believe, and therefore receive in Jesus' name. Amen!

"Casting all your care upon him; for he careth for you" (1 Peter 5:7).

Father, thank You for caring for me, therefore:
I cast all my worries on You.
I cast all my financial problems on You.
I cast all my family problems on You.
I cast burdens on You.
I cast my insecurities on You.
I cast low self-esteem on You.
I cast imposter syndrome on You.
I cast feeling inadequate on You.
I cast health problems on You.
I cast my "daddy" issues on You.
I cast my "mommy" issues on You.
I cast my business affairs on You.
I cast the care of my community on You.
I cast the care of my children on You.
I cast the care of the widows and orphans on You.
I cast the care of the sick on You who are in my sphere of influence.
I cast the care of the sin-sick on You who are in my sphere of influence.

"Casting down imaginations, and every high thing that exalteth itself against the knowledge of God, and bringing into captivity every thought to the obedience of Christ;" (2 Corinthians 10:5).

I pull down every thought that says I will never be healed.

I pull down every thought that says I will never be successful.

I pull down every thought that says that I will always be broke.

I pull down every thought that says we will always be poor.

I pull down every generational curse.

I pull down every manifestation from a generation curse.

I denounce every generational curse.

I come out of agreement with every word curse spoken over me.

I come out of agreement with every word curse that I have spoken over myself.

I denounce and come out of every word curse I have spoken over my family members.

I pull down every thought that says I will die of this disease.

I pull down every thought that says my children will inherit this disease.

I pull down every thought that says my children will not be successful.

I pull down every thought that says my children will not inherit the land you promised me.

I pull down every thought that says we are borrowers and not lenders.

I pull down every thought that says we are beneath and not above.

I pull down every thought that says we are not a delightsome land.

I pull down every thought that says that my storehouses are not full.

I pull down every thought that says my barns are not filled with plenty.

I pull down every thought that says I am not blessed in the city.

I pull down every thought that says I am not blessed in the field.

I pull down every thought that says I am not blessed with I come or when I go.

I pull down every thought that says that I will not live to see the goodness of the Lord in my generation.

"A good man out of the good treasure of his heart bringeth forth that which is good; and an evil man out of the evil treasure of his heart bringeth forth that which is evil: for of the abundance of the heart his mouth speaketh" (Luke 6:45).

My heart is full of good things; therefore, my mouth speaks them according to **Luke 6:45.**
My heart is full of the joy of the Lord.
My heart is full of abundant peace.
My heart is full of compassion for others.
My heart is full of words that build others up.
My heart is full of laughter; therefore, it is like medicine.
My heart is full of love, for God is love.
My heart is full of care for others.
My heart is full to the overflowing with goodness.
My heart is full to the overflowing with mercy.

"Wherefore seeing we also are compassed about with so great a cloud of witnesses, let us lay aside every weight, and the sin which doth so easily beset us, and let us run with patience the race that is set before us" (Hebrews 12:1).

Father, thank You for my heavenly cheering section. Thank You that they are cheering me on to finish the race strong. I repent for every sin, every thought that displeased you, and every action that was opposite of Your plan for me. I receive Your forgiveness so that I can finish the race that You have set before me in Jesus' name. Amen!

"For thou, Lord, wilt bless the righteous; with favour wilt thou compass him as with a shield" (Psalm 5:12).

Thank you, Father, for surrounding me with Your grace.

Thank You, Father, for surrounding me with Your mercy.

Thank You, Father, for surrounding me with Your love.

Thank You, Father, for surrounding me with Your peace.

Thank You, Father, for surrounding me with Your protection.

Thank You, Father, for surrounding me with Your light.

"Come unto me, all ye that labour and are heavy laden, and I will give you rest. Take my yoke upon you and learn of me; for I am meek and lowly in heart: and ye shall find rest unto your souls. For my yoke is easy, and my burden is light" (Matthew 11:28-30).

Father, thank you for your invitation to bring my burdens and cares to you. Thank you for a secure place to rest in you. Thank you for offering your gentle and humble heart in which I can find safety from all my fears and woes. In Jesus' name. Amen!

"In my distress I called upon the Lord, and cried unto my God: he heard my voice out of his temple, and my cry came before him, even into his ears" (Psalm 18:6).

I cried to my God for help with depression, and He heard me.

I cried to my God for help with oppression, and He heard me.

I cried to my God for help with low self-esteem, and He heard me.

I cried to my God for help with imposter syndrome, and He heard me.

I cried to my God for help with domestic violence, and He heard me.

I cried to my God for help with spousal abuse, and He heard me.

I cried to my God for help with child abuse, and He heard me.

I cried to my God for help with the generational curse, and He heard me.

I cried to my God for help with words curses that were spoken over me, and He heard me.

"And it shall come to pass in that day, that his burden shall be taken away from off thy shoulder, and his yoke from off thy neck, and the yoke shall be destroyed because of the anointing" (Isaiah 10:27).

I decree and declare according to **Isaiah 10:27** that the burden of poverty, the burden of lack, the burden of mental anguish, the burden of low self-esteem, the burden of not feeling good enough shall be off of my neck, and its yoke is broken off of me. In Jesus' name. Amen

"We are troubled on every side, yet not distressed; we are perplexed, but not in despair; Persecuted, but not forsaken; cast down, but not destroyed" (2 Corinthians 4:8-9).

Thank you, Father, regardless of the issues that come my way, I am not in despair, I am not abandoned, and I am not destroyed. Though I am pressed heard on every side, I still win. I still prosper, and I still succeed! In Jesus' name. Amen

"Though I walk in the midst of trouble, thou wilt revive me: thou shalt stretch forth thine hand against the wrath of mine enemies, and thy right hand shall save me" (Psalm 138:7)

God preserves my life by stretching His hand against generational curses that come to kill my life, to steal my life, to destroy my life. Thank you, Father, for saving me with Your right hand.

"Be careful for nothing; but in everything by prayer and supplication with thanksgiving let your requests be made known unto God. And the peace of God, which passeth all understanding, shall keep your hearts and minds through Christ Jesus" (Philippians 4:6-7).

I will not be anxious, afraid, and overwhelmed because I present my requests to God with thanksgiving; therefore, His peace gives me understanding and guards my heart and mind in Christ Jesus!

"When thou liest down, thou shalt not be afraid: yea, thou shalt lie down, and thy sleep shall be sweet" (Proverbs 3:24).

Because I have sought wisdom and understanding, I will lie down to sleep without fear, and my sleep will be sweet and trouble-free.

I rebuke sleeplessness.

I rebuke insomnia.

I rebuke night terrors.

I rebuke bad dreams.

I rebuke restlessness.

I rebuke tiredness that would inhibit my sleep.

I rebuke weariness.

I rebuke stress that would come to cause me to toss and turn.

I come again every spirit of infirmity that would try to take residence in my mind and rob me from sweet sleep.

I bind nervousness.

I bind anxiety.

I bind sleepwalking.

I bind sleep talking.

I bind overactive minds that won't allow for a restful, restorative sleep.

I loose creative and restorative sleep.

I loose sleep that is refreshing and supports innovative planning.

I loose sleep that causes me to sleep like a baby without a single care.

I loose sleep that allows me to rest well in the arms of the Father.

"He that dwelleth in the secret place of the Most High shall abide under the shadow of the Almighty. I will say of the Lord, He is my refuge and my fortress: my God; in him will I trust. Surely he shall deliver thee from the snare of the fowler, and from the noisome pestilence. He shall cover thee with his feathers, and under his wings shalt thou trust: his truth shall be thy shield and buckler. Thou shalt not be afraid for the terror by night; nor for the arrow that flieth by day; Nor for the pestilence that walketh in darkness; nor for the destruction that wasteth at noonday. A thousand shall fall at thy side, and ten thousand at thy right hand; but it shall not come nigh thee. Only with thine eyes shalt thou behold and see the reward of the wicked. Because thou hast made the Lord, which is my refuge, even the Most High, thy habitation; There shall no evil befall thee, neither shall any plague come nigh thy dwelling. For he shall give his angels charge over thee, to keep thee in all thy ways. They shall bear thee up in their hands, lest thou dash thy foot against a stone. Thou shalt tread upon the lion and adder: the young lion and the dragon shalt thou trample under feet. Because he hath set his love upon me, therefore will I deliver him: I will set him on high, because he hath known my name. He shall call upon me, and I will answer him: I will be with him in trouble; I will deliver him, and honour him. With long life will I satisfy him, and shew him my salvation" (Psalm 91).

Confess the power, authority, and protection of **Psalms 91**. Thank You, Father, for allowing me to rest in Your shadow and dwell in Your shelter. You, oh Lord, are my refuge, fortress, and the only God in whom I trust. Thank You for giving the angels charge over me, and they stand guard over me, making sure that I don't even stub my toe. Thank You for the power to walk on lions and snakes and not be harmed. Because I love and acknowledge Your great name, You rescue me, answer when I call, and are present with me in trouble. Thank You, Father, for showing Your salvation and giving me long life.

"The Spirit of the Lord God is upon me; because the Lord hath anointed me to preach good tidings unto the meek; he hath sent me to bind up the brokenhearted, to proclaim liberty to the captives, and the opening of the prison to them that are bound; To proclaim the acceptable year of the Lord, and the day of vengeance of our God; to comfort all that mourn; To appoint unto them that mourn in Zion, to give unto them beauty for ashes, the oil of joy for mourning, the garment of praise for the spirit of heaviness; that they might be called trees of righteousness, the planting of the Lord, that he might be glorified." (Isaiah 61:1-3)

Father, I thank You for the divine exchange that Your Good News has brought!
Thank You for binding my broken heart!
Thank You for setting me free when I was held captive and in prison to sin, despair, hopelessness, helplessness, depression, and oppression.!
Because of Your favor and vengeance, You comfort me when I mourn and grieve over the wrongs that I have done.
Because of Your favor, You crown me with beauty instead of ashes.
You anoint me with the oil of joy.
I dance before You in the garment of praise that You gave me instead of the despair that tried to hold me back.
I am grateful that I am called the oaks of righteousness, a tree planted by the rivers of water for Your glory and splendor.

Father, I thank you that according to **2 Corinthians 12:9:**
Your grace is sufficient for me when I am weak.
Your grace is sufficient for me when the enemy tries to discourage me.
Your grace is sufficient for me when the enemy tries to whisper lies about my future in my ears.
Your grace is sufficient for me when the enemy accuses me of the opposite of what Your Word says I am.
Your grace is sufficient for me when my body is not lining up when Your Word says. I am fearfully and wonderfully made.
Your grace is sufficient, for Your power is made perfect in my weakness.
Your power is made perfect when I feel weak.
Your power is made perfect when I feel frail and want to give up.
Your power is made perfect even when I fall for the lies and schemes of the enemy, but Your power comes to rescue me every time! Therefore, I will boast all the more gladly about my weaknesses so that Christ's power may rest on me!

"For my thoughts are not your thoughts, neither are your ways my ways, saith the Lord. For as the heavens are higher than the earth, so are my ways higher than your ways, and my thoughts than your thoughts" (Isaiah 55:8-9)

Father, I present Your Word to You, thank You for performing it. In Jesus' name. Amen.

"Let the words of my mouth, and the meditation of my heart, be acceptable in thy sight, O Lord, my strength, and my redeemer" (Psalm 19:14)

Father, I commit the speech and how I think to you that You be pleased with me. In the matchless name of Jesus Christ, the Anointed One and His Anointing!

Appendix B

"I Am the Church" Declarations and Confessions

- I am healed and healthy.

- My faith makes me whole.

- Because the Lord is my Shepherd, I lack nothing.

- The Lord cares for me.

- The Lord protects me.

- The Lord comforts me.

- The Lord gives me peace.

- The Lord blesses me.

- The Lord restores me.

- The Lord gives me rest.

- I am successful naturally and spiritually.

- I am prosperous naturally and spiritually.

- I am financially prosperous.

- I am a tither, so I live under an open heaven.

- I am in good health.

- I can give my issues to my Father because He cares for me.

- The Kingdom of God is in me.

- I love others as myself.

- I love others as God loves them.

- God loves me.

- I am healed by the stripes of Jesus.

- My peace was bought by Jesus.

- I am the head and not the tail.

- I am above only and not beneath.

- I am the Church.

- I am the Body of Christ.

- I was purchased by the blood of Jesus.

- I seek wisdom and understanding.

- I am a friend of God.

- I give my all for Christ.

- My faith is encouraging to others.

- Love fulfills the law.

- I am not judgmental.

- I am attached to the Vine.

- The name of the Lord is my Strong Tower.

- I have divine health.

- I am Abrahams's seed.

- My mind is renewed daily.

- The joy of the Lord is my strength.

- I am fearfully and wonderfully made by God.

- I am made in God's image.

- I lay aside every weight that could hold me back.

- I have the mind of Christ.

- I am more than a conqueror. Life and death are in my tongue; therefore, I speak life.

- God's favor overtakes me.

Appendix C

Personalized Prayers and Declarations

Fill in the blanks with your concerns, needs, and desires.

"Heal me, O Lord, and I shall be healed; save me, and I shall be saved: for thou art my praise" (Jeremiah 17:14).

Father, you are my praise! Thank You for healing my _____.

"And ye shall serve the Lord your God, and he shall bless thy bread, and thy water; and I will take sickness away from the midst of thee" (Exodus 23:25).

Because I serve the Lord, He blesses me and has removed _____ from me!

"Fear thou not; for I am with thee: be not dismayed; for I am thy God: I will strengthen thee; yea, I will help thee; yea, I will uphold thee with the right hand of my righteousness" (Isaiah 41:10).

ThankYou,Fatherfordeliveringmefromthefearof_____.
ThankYou,Fatherfordeliveringmefromthefearof_____.
ThankYou,Fatherfordeliveringmefromthefearof_____.
ThankYou,Fatherfordeliveringmefromthefearof_____.
ThankYou,Fatherfordeliveringmefromthefearof_____.

"For I will restore health unto thee, and I will heal thee of thy wounds, saith the Lord; because they called thee an Outcast, saying, This is Zion, whom no man seeketh after" (Jeremiah 30:17).

Father, thank You for caring for me when others called me an outcast.
Thank You for restoring my _____ health and healing my _____ wounds.
Thank You for restoring my _____ health and healing my _____ wounds.
Thank You for restoring my _____ health and healing my _____ wounds.
Thank You for restoring my _____ health and healing my _____ wounds.

"But my God shall supply all your need according to his riches in glory by Christ Jesus" (Philippians 4:19).

According to Philippians 4:19, I walk in a liberal supply of _____.

According to Philippians 4:19, I walk in a liberal supply of _____.

According to Philippians 4:19, I walk in a liberal supply of _____.

According to Philippians 4:19, I walk in a liberal supply of _____.

According to Philippians 4:19, I walk in a liberal supply of _____.

Thank You, Father, that this supply is based on Your riches in glory in Jesus Christ, the anointing One, and His anointing!

"Pleasant words are as an honeycomb, sweet to the soul, and health to the bones" (Proverbs 16:24).

Father, please let the words of my mouth and the meditation of my heart be acceptable in Thy sight. Let them be sweet and pleasing. Let them be kind and uplifting. Let them be tasty and delightful so that body may be healed.

"He healeth the broken in heart, and bindeth up their wounds" (Psalms 147:3).

Father, in the name of Jesus, someone reading this has a heart that has been wounded through abuse from the one who was supposed to love them, the one who was supposed to support them, who was supposed to protect them. This abuse has caused them to walk around with weeping wounds. They bleed on others because they are hurt, and hurting people hurt others. They don't want to be this way, but their gaping wounds have festered and become infected. It has caused stinking thinking about not only others but about themselves as well. They have internalized the things that were said to them, and now they believe that they are what was placed on them spiritually. You said in **Psalms 147:13** that You heal the brokenhearted. Thank You, Father, for performing a heart transplant on them now. Out of the heart flows the issues of life. Re-center, re-direct, and restore them for Your Kingdom's sake. Thank You for wrapping them up in Your love as You bind their wounds. Hold them tight, Father, so that they can feel Your heartbeat. So that they can experience Your love with every beat. Thank You for giving them beauty for ashes, oil of joy for mourning, and the garment of praise for the spirit of heaviness. Please give laughter as medicine and peace like a river. In Jesus' name!

"And the Lord shall guide thee continually, and satisfy thy soul in drought, and make fat thy bones: and thou shalt be like a watered garden, and like a spring of water, whose waters fail not" (Isaiah 58:11).

Father, according to Your Word in **Isaiah 58:11,** we look to you for continual guidance, thank You for water the dry and cracked places of _____ in my life. Please send a deluge of water from the fountain of your love and healing that will spring up in those areas causing them to be a well-watered garden. We will then pluck the beautiful roses and flowers that grow in this now healthy place and distribute them freely as You have given them freely to us as You lead in Jesus' name.

"How God anointed Jesus of Nazareth with the Holy Ghost and with power: who went about doing good, and healing all that were oppressed of the devil; for God was with him" (Acts 10:38).

Thank You, Father for healing these areas of oppression in my life _____. Thank You, Jesus, for the power You possess to heal these areas. I receive this healing. I come out of agreement with every word and deed that was sent to hold me down, to oppress me, and to suppress me. I repent for agreeing with the word curses that were spoken over me because I didn't realize and believe who I was in You. I decree and declare that the devil no longer has the legal right to block me from being all that You have called me to be. I decree and declare that I am loosed from the infirmity of oppression in my mind, in my spirit, in my heart. I decree and declare that I am free from every negative thought that would attempt to exalt itself the knowledge that You are ruler and King in my life, and therefore I pull down every high thing that would come to try to stifle me. Thank You for the liberty that Christ died to give me in Jesus' name!

"Then shall thy light break forth as the morning, and thine health shall spring forth speedily: and thy righteousness shall go before thee; the glory of the Lord shall be thy reward" (Isaiah 58:8).

Then (insert your name) light will break out like the dawn, and (insert your name) healing (name it) (restoration, new life) will quickly spring forth; (insert your name) righteousness will go before (insert him or her) [leading (insert your name) to peace and prosperity], the glory of the Lord will be (insert your name) rear guard. Thank You, Lord! In Jesus' name!

Citations

1. World Health Organization. About World Health Organization. Constitution. Available at: http://www.who.int/governance/eb/constitution/en/

2. Sohn-Kahn, JaneSara (June 2020). https://www.healthpopuli.com/2020/06/19/juneteenth-2020-inequality-and-injustice-in-health-care-in-america

3. https://www.cdc.gov/chronicdisease/about/index.htm (last reviewed 4/28/2021)

4. http://kingjamesbibledictionary.com/StrongsNo/H4437/kingdom

5. https://www.Brittannica.com/science/disease

6. https://www.merriam-webster.com/dictionary/dis

7. https://www.merriam-webster.com/dictionary/ease

8. https://www.biblestudytools.com/lexicons/greek/nas/ekklesia.html

9. https://www.merriam-webster.com/dictionary/healthcare

10. https://dictionary.com/care

11. History of Healthy People Initiative https://health.gov/our-work/healthy-people/about-healthy-people/history-healthy-people

12. 2000 Healthy People Final Report https://www.cdc.gov/nchs/data/hp2000/hp2k01/p.6.pdf

13. http://www.usachurches.org/church-sizes.htm

14. https://www.merriam-webster.com/dictionary/impartation

15. Olshansky SJ, Antonucci T, Berkman L, Binstock RH, Boersch-Supan A, Cacioppo JT, Carnes BA, Carstensen LL, Fried LP, Goldman DP, Jackson J, Kohli M, Rother J, Zheng Y, Rowe J. Differences in life expectancy due to race and educational

differences are widening, and many may not catch up. Health Aff (Millwood). 2012 Aug;31(8):1803-13. doi: 10.1377/hlthaff.2011.0746. PMID: 22869659.

16. https://www.valamis.com/hub/adult-learning-principles

17. https://www.churchleadership.com/wp-content/uploads/2017/10/50-Ways-to-Strengthen-Adult-Education.pdf

18. https://www.everydayhealth.com/mens-health/ways-stress-affects-mens-health.aspx

19. Megan L. Evans, M.D., M.P.H., Margo Lindauer, J.D., and Maureen E. Farrell, M.D. N Engl J Med 2020; A Pandemic within a Pandemic — Intimate Partner Violence during Covid-19 383:2302-2304 DOI: 10.1056/NEJMp2024046

20. Fernando, Jason. https://www.investopedia.com/terms/f/financial-literacy.asp

21. https://www.psychiatry.org/patients-families/what-is-mental-illness

22. https://www.nimh.nih.gov/health/statistics/mental-illness

23. https://www.psychiatry.org/File%20Library/Psychiatrists/Cultural-Competency/faith-mentalhealth-guide.pdf

24. https://www.christianitytoday.com/pastors/2016/april-web-exclusives/top-10-resources-for-mental-health-ministry.html

25. https://www.resourceumc.org/en/content/resources-for-mental-health-ministries

Resource Sites

- https://www.chihealth.com
- https://www.faithandhealthconnection.org
- https://store.churchhealth.org
- https://Health.gov

Observances and National Health Awareness Days

- National Childhood Obesity Awareness Month
- National Recovery Month
- National Breast and Cervical Cancer Early Detection Program
- National Stalking Awareness Month
- American Heart Month
- National Wear Red Day
- Women's Health Month
- National Women and Girls HIV/AIDS Awareness Day
- American Stroke Month
- Healthy Aging Month
- National Diabetes Month

About The Author

Phyllis Carter-Riles, RN, "the Kingdom nurse," is the founder of Phyllis C. Riles LLC. Through her consulting firm Phyllis C. Riles Consulting, Phyllis has dedicated her life and career to sharing her healthcare knowledge with people across various sectors, including the Church. Her love for God's people and her passion for teaching prompted the formation of the *Rapha Health Ministry* at her church. This program with an adaptable curriculum became the avenue through which she has launched many health events and programs developed to usher people into prosperous, healthy lives.

A devoted, lifelong learner, Phyllis has utilized her Nursing and Health Administration degrees along with other advanced certifications—including the coveted Certification in Infection Control (CIC)—to promote health through innovative and insightful topics. Voted the *Kingdom Business Network (KBN)* 2021 *World Leader of the Year* and Motivator of the year, exhibiting another characteristic of the Church, Phyllis seeks opportunities to help others achieve health and wholeness through natural strategies and Biblical principles.

Phyllis lives in Texas with her husband James, their adult children, seven grandchildren, and "fur girl" Ginger. To learn more about Phyllis and the educational or consulting services she provides, please visit www.phylliscrilesconsulting.com.

www.ingramcontent.com/pod-product-compliance
Lightning Source LLC
Chambersburg PA
CBHW071135280326
41935CB00010B/1231